T0092088

What's in the Syringe?

What's in the Syringe?

Principles of Early Integrated Palliative Care

JULIET JACOBSEN, MD
MEDICAL DIRECTOR FOR THE CONTINUUM PROJECT
ASSOCIATE PROFESSOR OF MEDICINE, HARVARD MEDICAL SCHOOL
DEPARTMENT OF MEDICINE, DIVISION OF PALLIATIVE CARE AND GERIATRIC MEDICINE
MASSACHUSETTS GENERAL HOSPITAL
BOSTON, MA, USA

VICKI JACKSON, MD, MPH
CHIEF, DIVISION OF PALLIATIVE CARE AND GERIATRIC MEDICINE
CO-DIRECTOR, HARVARD MEDICAL SCHOOL CENTER FOR PALLIATIVE CARE
ASSOCIATE PROFESSOR OF MEDICINE, HARVARD MEDICAL SCHOOL
DEPARTMENT OF MEDICINE
MASSACHUSETTS GENERAL HOSPITAL
HARVARD MEDICAL SCHOOL
BOSTON, MA, USA

JOSEPH GREER, PHD
CO-DIRECTOR, CANCER OUTCOMES RESEARCH AND EDUCATION PROGRAM
PROGRAM DIRECTOR, CENTER FOR PSYCHIATRIC ONCOLOGY AND
BEHAVIORAL SCIENCES
ASSOCIATE PROFESSOR OF PSYCHOLOGY, HARVARD MEDICAL SCHOOL
DEPARTMENT OF PSYCHIATRY
MASSACHUSETTS GENERAL HOSPITAL
BOSTON, MA, USA

JENNIFER TEMEL, MD
CO-DIRECTOR, CANCER OUTCOMES RESEARCH AND EDUCATION PROGRAM
CLINICAL DIRECTOR, THORACIC ONCOLOGY
PROFESSOR OF MEDICINE, HARVARD MEDICAL SCHOOL
DEPARTMENT OF MEDICINE, DIVISION OF HEMATOLOGY/ONCOLOGY
MASSACHUSETTS GENERAL HOSPITAL
BOSTON, MA, USA

OXFORD
UNIVERSITY PRESS

OXFORD
UNIVERSITY PRESS

Oxford University Press is a department of the University of Oxford. It furthers
the University's objective of excellence in research, scholarship, and education
by publishing worldwide. Oxford is a registered trade mark of Oxford University
Press in the UK and certain other countries.

Published in the United States of America by Oxford University Press
198 Madison Avenue, New York, NY 10016, United States of America.

© Oxford University Press 2021

All rights reserved. No part of this publication may be reproduced, stored in
a retrieval system, or transmitted, in any form or by any means, without the
prior permission in writing of Oxford University Press, or as expressly permitted
by law, by license, or under terms agreed with the appropriate reproduction
rights organization. Inquiries concerning reproduction outside the scope of the
above should be sent to the Rights Department, Oxford University Press, at the
address above.

You must not circulate this work in any other form
and you must impose this same condition on any acquirer.

Library of Congress Cataloging-in-Publication Data
Names: Jacobsen, Juliet, author. | Jackson, Vicki A., 1968– author. |
Greer, Joseph A., author. | Temel, Jennifer, author.
Title: What's in the syringe? : principles of early integrated palliative
care / Juliet Jacobsen, Vicki Jackson, Joseph Greer, and Jennifer Temel.
Description: New York, NY : Oxford University Press, [2021] | Includes
bibliographical references and index.
Identifiers: LCCN 2021009995 (print) | LCCN 2021009996 (ebook) |
ISBN 9780197525173 (paperback) | ISBN 9780197525197 (epub) |
ISBN 9780197525203 (online)
Subjects: MESH: Palliative Care—psychology | Integrative
Oncology—psychology | Physician-Patient Relations | Patient Care Management
Classification: LCC R726.8 (print) | LCC R726.8 (ebook) | NLM WB 310 |
DDC 616.02/9—dc23
LC record available at https://lccn.loc.gov/2021009995
LC ebook record available at https://lccn.loc.gov/2021009996

DOI: 10.1093/med/9780197525173.001.0001

This material is not intended to be, and should not be considered, a substitute for medical or other
professional advice. Treatment for the conditions described in this material is highly dependent on
the individual circumstances. And, while this material is designed to offer accurate information with
respect to the subject matter covered and to be current as of the time it was written, research and
knowledge about medical and health issues is constantly evolving and dose schedules for medications
are being revised continually, with new side effects recognized and accounted for regularly. Readers
must therefore always check the product information and clinical procedures with the most up-to-date
published product information and data sheets provided by the manufacturers and the most recent
codes of conduct and safety regulation. The publisher and the authors make no representations or
warranties to readers, express or implied, as to the accuracy or completeness of this material. Without
limiting the foregoing, the publisher and the authors make no representations or warranties as to the
accuracy or efficacy of the drug dosages mentioned in the material. The authors and the publisher do
not accept, and expressly disclaim, any responsibility for any liability, loss, or risk that may be claimed
or incurred as a consequence of the use and/or application of any of the contents of this material.

To the memory of J. Andrew Billings (1945–2015)
Pioneer in Palliative Care

and

Founding Director of the Palliative Care Service
at Massachusetts General Hospital

CONTENTS

Most clinicians whom I know agree that the hardest work in palliative care is in communication and psychological care of patients. Although success in these endeavors often looks like magic, it is not. It is the application of competencies in symptom management and psychological assessment; relationship building; helping the patient tolerate strong and often oscillating emotions; teaching coping skills; titrating discussions to enhance prognostic awareness within tolerable limits; and shared decision-making. It requires that clinicians develop self-awareness and tolerate and manage their own strong emotions. These learnable competencies are not generally taught in medical school, residency, or most palliative care fellowships. Fortunately, this marvelous book provides a framework that demystifies and deconstructs what happens in successful palliative care relationships with patients, families, and colleagues, and it explicates how these competencies can be practiced in palliative care.

The field of palliative care was electrified in 2010 when the Massachusetts General Hospital (MGH)'s randomized controlled trial of early palliative care intervention was published in the *New England Journal of Medicine* and demonstrated, in palliative care patients, reduced rates of depression, improved quality of life, greater prognostic awareness, higher quality of care, and prolonged survival, when compared to other oncology patients. We finally had strong evidence that palliative care "worked" in cancer patients. Indeed, many of us joked ruefully that, if palliative care were a drug that demonstrated such positive results, everyone with cancer would be on it within a month. Then the questions arose: What aspects of palliative care contributed to improvements in quality of life and survival? What allowed the MGH team to achieve such results? Could other palliative care teams achieve the same results with their early intervention programs? How could it be accomplished?

The MGH program, begun in 1995, was established by my late husband Andy Billings, one of the pioneers in palliative care in the United States. When he started the program, Andy had already been a community-based primary care physician and hospice physician for 20 years and had done extensive training and work in the areas of the doctor–patient relationship, communication, ethics, medical education, hospice, and psychological care of medically ill patients. He brought these sensibilities to how he cared for and taught about patients. He had strong and clear values about the importance of psychosocial factors in caring for patients with serious illness. He thought critically about the complex ethical issues that arise in palliative care. He taught others to question assumptions and to ask uncomfortable questions. Because of Andy's leadership, his role modeling, and his commitment as an educator, these perspectives and values pervaded the MGH program from its inception and created a culture that valued and practiced expert psychological care of patients. Andy's vision, his value system about the importance of the doctor–patient relationship, his capacity to ask deep questions, and his commitment to patients ground the work described in this book. His early ideas and values have been elaborated, expanded, and enhanced by the next generation of palliative care clinicians, researchers, and educators.

The authors of this book have created a relationally oriented synthesis of the theory and practice of high-quality care for seriously ill patients and their families. In addition, they use the same relational framework to describe collaborating with other clinicians and attending to their perspectives and emotions. Michael Balint, the author of what I think Andy would say was the medical book that had the deepest influence on him, wrote about "the drug, the doctor," and sought to deconstruct the active ingredients of the doctor–patient relationship that are healing for sick persons. This book is in that tradition. The book expands the idea of the "doctor–patient relationship" to include the whole clinical team caring for the patient. It describes how team members can collaborate with and support each other and how clinicians can use evidence-based constructs to help patients and families negotiate the experience of a serious illness in a "psychologically informed" manner.

Andy would be immensely proud of this work.

Susan Block, MD
Founding Chair Emerita, Department of Psychosocial
Oncology and Palliative Care
Dana-Farber Cancer Institute and Brigham and Women's Hospital
Founding Director (with Andy Billings) Emerita
Harvard Medical School Center for Palliative Care
Professor of Psychiatry and Medicine
Harvard Medical School

PURPOSE OF THIS BOOK

In 2003, Massachusetts General Hospital (MGH), a leading U.S. academic hospital, began offering palliative care to outpatients with metastatic cancer. The care started at the time of diagnosis of metastatic disease and ran concurrently with outpatient cancer care. In a traditional inpatient model, palliative care is usually initiated later in the course of disease, when a patient deteriorates medically or struggles with significant symptoms or the stress of a serious illness. Now not limited to cancer patients, early integrated palliative care begins near the diagnosis of advanced disease and continues throughout disease progression. Because this type of palliative care can last for months or years, it provides continuity for patients, families, and clinicians.

Over many years, our team has developed a specific approach to the clinical delivery and teaching of early integrated palliative care. The approach, unique and not yet a part of traditional palliative care training, is based on more than a decade of research and clinical experience. This book, a "how to" guide for clinicians and program leaders considering the approach, explains the approach, its rationale, and the research that informs it.

HOW WE DEVELOPED THIS APPROACH

We developed this approach because we worried about our patients, especially those with cancers of the lung and pancreas who often had a
poor prognosis. From the time of diagnosis, these patients had significant symptoms and distress. They were often unprepared for living with
serious illness and for end-of-life decision-making. But we didn't know
whether early integrated palliative care would be acceptable to them or
their oncologists.

As an experiment to address the unmet palliative care needs of these
patients, oncologist Jennifer Temel and palliative care clinicians Andy
Billings, Coleen Reid, Vicki Jackson, and Constance Dahlin built an outpatient palliative care program. The program would offer palliative care to
outpatients early in the illness trajectory and integrate it with cancer care.

The study of this approach began with feasibility: Would oncologists
enroll their patients with newly diagnosed disease in early integrated palliative care? Some oncologists worried that earlier palliative care involve-
ment might stress patients and families and perhaps worsen outcomes.
Patients might even give up and die sooner. In the feasibility study, we also
hoped to learn whether patients would participate in palliative care visits.

In the study, we saw how, as palliative care clinicians, we could
help these patients. We helped them manage the side effects of first
treatments. We helped them incorporate treatment into their lives and
cope with stress. We also helped them think about the future. Because
we worked with them for many months—and sometimes years—we
understood their goals and concerns. As their cancers progressed, we
could manage emerging symptoms and support them through medical
decision-making. Our work improved the experience of serious illness
for many patients.

Seeing that our model was feasible and acceptable to patients and
clinicians, we designed a randomized trial of early integrated palliative
care versus usual care for patients with newly diagnosed metastatic non-
small-cell lung cancer. Our goal was to test our preliminary impressions
that we were helping patients.

Fortunately, the primary results, published in 2010, confirmed our impressions. Early integrated palliative care had a significant impact. Patients randomly assigned to the intervention reported improved quality of life and had lower rates of depression compared to those who received usual oncology care alone. They had more accurate prognostic awareness, received higher-quality end-of-life care, and even lived longer. This study has become one of the most influential in palliative care.

Further research, including a Cochrane systematic review, has confirmed the beneficial clinical outcomes of early integrated palliative care. These positive results have had a broad impact. Professional organizations such as the American Society of Clinical Oncology now recommend considering referral to palliative care early in the course of disease for patients with metastatic cancer.

Through these initial studies, we had learned *that* this model of integrating palliative care with oncology works. But how did it work? As hospitals and cancer clinics across the country began to implement this early integrated model, clinicians and researchers began asking us, "What's in the syringe?" To answer this question and refine our understanding, we studied our palliative care practice. We conducted focus groups with the palliative care clinicians who served as study interventionists to tease out the different and sometimes competing roles of the palliative care clinician. We also studied what happens during our clinical care. As part of a larger follow-up trial of the early integrated palliative care model, we reviewed study patient charts and collected data about our clinical interventions. To understand the subtleties of what clinicians say, we made audio recordings of our intervention visits with patients. Extracts from these conversations appear as illustrative examples throughout the book.

WHAT WE LEARNED

We learned how we help patients live well with serious illness: We do so by managing symptoms, aggressively when needed, and by teaching patients skills to cope. It is a given that symptom assessment and management are essential to palliative care. However, survey data from patients and clinicians across thousands of study visits showed us that early integrated palliative care improves patients' quality of life and mood through enhancing their coping skills. These skills help patients to manage distressing thoughts and feelings and thereby to make the most of their time. Few patients have developed the breadth of coping skills required to face life-limiting illness. As one said, "I've never died before." Thus, a central theme of this book is how clinicians can help patients learn and use these skills.

Our approach to teaching coping skills includes ongoing discussions about how to live well with serious illness, in whatever ways that living well is defined by the patient. It also includes discussions about coping with worries, so that they do not interfere with living fully. Coping with worries also helps patients to prepare for end of life. In particular, patients must learn to cope with their deepening prognostic awareness: with their understanding of their most likely timeframe and illness trajectory. Coping effectively with this understanding helps patients plan and make informed end-of-life decisions. Most importantly, it helps patients live well throughout the illness.

Understandably, however, many patients resist conversations about the future and struggle to adapt to their prognosis. Integrating one's mortality with hopes to live longer is a difficult process that needs time. This hard work of coping with serious illness requires impeccable symptom management, so that patients feel well enough to engage in these discussions.

Although symptom management protocols are not the focus of this book, we do discuss how symptom management is a part of clinical attunement, a term we use that reflects the clinician's responsiveness to patients' needs in the setting of serious illness (this term is discussed throughout the book). As much as titrating opioids, clinical attunement is fundamental to our role as clinicians. By being attuned to patients' symptom and coping needs, we improve their quality of life, which gives patients greater capacity to more deeply understand their prognosis and reflect on their priorities. We also build a trusting relationship that helps us guide shared decision-making and enables patients, during their most difficult times, to trust our guidance.

Our approach was developed with cancer patients, but we have found that many of the underlying principles of clinical care also transfer to other illnesses such as heart or lung disease. Our approach was also developed with a largely White, English-speaking population, but patients from diverse cultures and backgrounds are included in our research and clinical care. In our experience, when clinicians understand the disease trajectory, are sensitive to information preferences, and can engage in shared decision-making, they provide individualized medical care that accords with patients' needs, culture, and background.

HOW THIS BOOK IS ORGANIZED

We have conceptualized our clinical approach as five challenges through which the clinician guides the patient (Figure 0.1). As patients take up each challenge, they build their capacity for the next and for living and dying well. (Although these challenges are taken up roughly linearly, patients may move back and forth as they build needed capacities and may even be struggling with multiple challenges simultaneously.) The five challenges draw from dialectical behavioral therapy (DBT) and acceptance

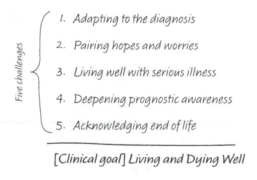

Figure 0.1. Five challenges facing patients with serious illness

and commitment therapy (ACT). These therapies teach acceptance, distress tolerance, and awareness to help people live with painful realities, including cancer. Taking up these challenges, patients learn to live in a healthy dialectic between seemingly contradictory ideas: living well and acknowledging end of life.

The chapters in the book address the challenges in roughly the order that they occur in the disease trajectory. Chapters 1 and 2 address challenges that patients face soon after diagnosis. Chapters 3 and 4 address challenges from the middle of the illness trajectory. Chapter 5 addresses the challenge that comes with disease progression. Each chapter offers clinicians an approach grounded in our research and clinical experience. Each includes communication skills to help patients with the challenge and strategies to support their coping.

In each chapter, we also discuss how oncologists and palliative care clinicians can collaborate most effectively. Our research and clinical work have taught us that early integrated palliative care has to be collaborative. Palliative care clinicians often facilitate communication between the oncologist and the patient and therefore need to understand the complexity of their own role in the medical team. We also discuss potential conflicts between oncologists and palliative care clinicians and share strategies for resolution, so that we can together support patients through serious illness.

What is in the syringe of early integrated palliative care? It is the collaborative effort by palliative care and oncology clinicians to help patients and families live well with serious illness by taking up the following five challenges.

SELECTED REFERENCES FOR OUR TEAM'S RESEARCH

Back, A. L., Park, E. R., Greer, J. A., Jackson, V. A., Jacobsen, J. C., Gallagher, E. R., & Temel, J. S. (2014). Clinician roles in early integrated palliative care for patients with advanced cancer: A qualitative study. *Journal of Palliative Medicine*, *17*(11), 1244–1248.

Bickel, K. E., Levy, C., MacPhee, E. R., Brenner, K., Temel, J. S., Arch, J. A., & Greer, J. A. (2020). An integrative framework of appraisal and adaptation in serious medical illness. *Journal of Pain and Symptom Management*, *60*(3), 657–677.

El-Jawahri, A., Forst, D., Fenech, A., Brenner, K. O., Jankowski, A. L., Waldman, L., Sereno, I., Nipp, R., Greer, J. A., Traeger, L., Jackson, V., & Temel, J. (2020). Relationship between perceptions of treatment goals and psychological distress in patients with advanced cancer. *Journal of the National Comprehensive Cancer Network, 18*(7), 849–855.

El-Jawahri, A., Greer, J. A., Pirl, W. F., Park, E. R., Jackson, V. A., Back, A. L., Kamdar, M., Jacobsen, J., Chittenden, E. H., Rinaldi, S. P., Gallagher, E. R., Eusebio, J. R., Fishman, S., VanDusen, H., Li, Z., Muzikansky, A., & Temel, J. S. (2017). Effects of early integrated palliative care on caregivers of patients with lung and gastrointestinal cancer: A randomized clinical trial. *The Oncologist, 22*(12), 1528–1534.

Ferrell, B. R., Temel, J. S., Temin, S., Alesi, E. R., Balboni, T. A., Basch, E. M., Firn, J. I., Paice, J. A., Peppercorn, J. M., Phillips, T., Stovall, E. L., Zimmermann, C., & Smith, T. J. (2017). Integration of palliative care into standard oncology care: American Society of Clinical Oncology clinical practice guideline update. *Journal of Clinical Oncology, 35*(1), 96–112.

Fujisawa, D., Temel, J. S., Traeger, L., Greer, J. A., Lennes, I. T., Mimura, M., & Pirl, W. F. (2015). Psychological factors at early stage of treatment as predictors of receiving chemotherapy at the end of life. *Psycho-oncology, 24*(12), 1731–1737.

Fulton, J. J., LeBlanc, T. W., Cutson, T. M., Porter Starr, K. N., Kamal, A., Ramos, K., Freiermuth, C. E., McDuffie, J. R., Kosinski, A., Adam, S., Nagi, A., & Williams, J. W. (2019). Integrated outpatient palliative care for patients with advanced cancer: A systematic review and meta-analysis. *Palliative Medicine, 33*(2), 123–134.

Greer, J. A., Applebaum, A. J., Jacobsen, J. C., Temel, J. A., & Jackson, V. A. (2020). Understanding and addressing the role of coping in palliative care for patients with advanced cancer. *Journal of Clinical Oncology, 38*(9), 915–25.

Greer, J. A., Jacobs, J. M., El-Jawahri, A., Nipp, R. D., Gallagher, E. R., Pirl, W. F., Park, E. R., Muzikansky, A., Jacobsen, J. C., Jackson, V. A., & Temel, J. S. (2018). Role of patient coping strategies in understanding the effects of early palliative care on quality of life and mood. *Journal of Clinical Oncology, 36*(1), 53–60.

Greer, J. A., Pirl, W. F., Jackson, V. A., Muzikansky, A., Lennes, I. T., Gallagher, E. R., Prigerson, H. G., & Temel, J. S. (2014). Perceptions of health status and survival in patients with metastatic lung cancer. *Journal of Pain and Symptom Management, 48*(4), 548–557.

Greer, J. A., Pirl, W. F., Jackson, V. A., Muzikansky, A., Lennes, I. T., Heist, R. S., Gallagher, E. R., & Temel, J. S. (2012). Effect of early palliative care on chemotherapy use and end-of-life care in patients with metastatic non-small-cell lung cancer. *Journal of Clinical Oncology, 30*(4), 394–400.

Greer, J. A., Tramontano, A. C., McMahon, P. M., Pirl, W. F., Jackson, V. A., El-Jawahri, A., Parikh, R. B., Muzikansky, A., Gallagher, E. R., & Temel, J. S. (2016). Cost analysis of a randomized trial of early palliative care in patients with metastatic non-small-cell lung cancer. *Journal of Palliative Medicine, 19*(8), 842–848.

Hagan, T. L., Fishbein, J. N., Nipp, R. D., Jacobs, J. M., Traeger, L., Irwin, K. E., Pirl, W. F., Greer, J. A., Park, E. R., Jackson, V. A., & Temel, J. S. (2017). Coping in patients with incurable lung and gastrointestinal cancers: A validation study of the Brief Cope. *Journal of Pain and Symptom Management, 53*(1), 131–138.

Haun, M. W., Estel, S., Rucker, G., Friederich, H. C., Villalobos, M., Thomas, M., & Hartmann, M. (2017). Early palliative care for adults with advanced cancer. *Cochrane Database of Systematic Reviews, 6*(6), CD011129.

Hoerger, M., Greer, J. A., Jackson, V. A., Park, E. R., Pirl, W. F., El-Jawahri, A., Gallagher, E. R., Hagan, T., Jacobsen, J., Perry, L. M., & Temel, J. S. (2018). Defining the elements of early palliative care that are associated with patient-reported outcomes and the delivery of end-of-life care. *Journal of Clinical Oncology, 36*(11), 1096–1102.

Irwin, K. E., Greer, J. A., Khatib, J., Temel, J. S., & Pirl, W. F. (2013). Early palliative care and metastatic non-small cell lung cancer: Potential mechanisms of prolonged survival. *Chronic Respiratory Disease, 10*(1), 35–47.

Jackson, V. A., Jacobsen, J. C., Greer, J., Dahlin, C., Billings, J. A., Pirl, E., Perez Cruz, W. P., Admane, S., Blinderman, C., & Temel, J. (2009). Components of early intervention outpatient palliative care consultation in patients with incurable NSCLC. *Journal of Clinical Oncology, 27*(15 Suppl), 459–464.

Jackson, V. A., Jacobsen, J. A., Greer, J. A., Pirl, W. F., Temel, J. S., & Back, A. L. (2013). Cultivation of prognostic awareness through the provision of early palliative care in the ambulatory setting: A communication guide. *Journal of Palliative Medicine, 16*(8), 894–900.

Jacobs, J. M., Shaffer, K. M., Nipp, R. D., Fishbein, J. N., MacDonald, J., El-Jawahri, A., Pirl, W. F., Jackson, V. A., Park, E. R., Temel, J. S., & Greer, J. A. (2017). Distress is interdependent in patients and caregivers with newly diagnosed incurable cancers. *Annals of Behavioral Medicine, 51*(4), 519–531.

Jacobsen, J., Jackson, V., Dahlin, C., Greer, J., Perez-Cruz, P., Billings, J. A., Pirl, W., & Temel, J. (2011). Components of early outpatient palliative care consultation in patients with metastatic non-small cell lung cancer. *Journal of Palliative Medicine, 14*(4), 459–464.

Jacobsen, J., Kvale, E., Rabow, M., Rinaldi, S., Cohen, S., Weissman, D., & Jackson, V. (2014). Helping patients with serious illness live well through the promotion of adaptive coping: A report from the Improving Outpatient Palliative Care (IPAL-OP) initiative. *Journal of Palliative Medicine, 17*(4), 463–468.

Nipp, R. D., El-Jawahri, A., Fishbein, J. N., Eusebio, J., Stagl, J. M., Gallagher, E. R., Park, E. R., Jackson, V. A., Pirl, W. F., Greer, J. A., & Temel, J. S. (2016). The relationship between coping strategies, quality of life, and mood in patients with incurable cancer. *Cancer, 122*(13), 2110–2116.

Nipp, R. D., El-Jawahri, A., Fishbein, J. N., Gallagher, E. R., Stagl, J. M., Park, E. R., Jackson, V. A., Pirl, W. F., Greer, J. A., & Temel, J. S. (2016). Factors associated with depression and anxiety symptoms in family caregivers of patients with incurable cancer. *Annals of Oncology, 27*(8), 1607–1612.

Nipp, R. D., El-Jawahri, A., Traeger, L., Jacobs, J. M., Gallagher, E. R., Park, E. R., Jackson, V. A., Pirl, W. F., Temel, J. S., & Greer, J. A. (2018). Differential effects of early palliative care based on the age and sex of patients with advanced cancer from a randomized controlled trial. *Palliative Medicine, 32*(4), 757–766.

Nipp, R., Greer, J., El-Jawahri, A., Moran, S., Traeger, L., Jacobs, J., Jacobsen, J., Gallagher, E. R., Park, E. R., Ryan, D. P., Jackson, V. A., Pirl, W. F., & Temel, J. S. (2017). Coping and prognostic awareness in patients with advanced cancer. *Journal of Clinical Oncology, 35*(22), 2551–2557.

Nipp, R. D., Greer, J. A., El-Jawahri, A., Traeger, L., Gallagher, E. R., Park, E. R., Jackson, V. A., Pirl, W. F., & Temel, J. S. (2016). Age and gender moderate the impact of early palliative care in metastatic non-small cell lung cancer. *Oncologist, 21*(1), 119–126.

Pirl, W. F., Greer, J. A., Irwin, K., Lennes, I. T., Jackson, V. A., Park, E. R., Fujisawa, D., Wright, A. A., & Temel, J. S. (2015). Processes of discontinuing chemotherapy for metastatic non-small-cell lung cancer at the end of life. *Journal of Oncology Practice, 11*(3), e405–e412.

Pirl, W. F., Greer, J. A., Traeger, L., Jackson, V., Lennes, I. T., Gallagher, E. R., Perez-Cruz, P., Heist, R. S., & Temel, J. S. (2012). Depression and survival in metastatic non-small-cell lung cancer: Effects of early palliative care. *Journal of Clinical Oncology, 30*(12), 1310–1315.Temel, J. S., Greer, J. A., Admane, S., Gallagher, E. R., Jackson, V. A., Lynch, T. J., Lennes, I. T., Dahlin, C. M., & Pirl, W. F. (2011). Longitudinal perceptions of prognosis and goals of therapy in patients with metastatic non-small-cell lung cancer: Results of a randomized study of early palliative care. *Journal of Clinical Oncology, 29*(17), 2319–2326.

Temel, J. S., Greer, J. A., El-Jawahir, A., Pirl, W. F., Park, E. R., Jackson, V. A., Back, A. L., Kamdar, M., Jacobsen, J., Chittenden, E. H., Rindaldi, S. P., Gallagher, E. R., Eusebio, J. R., Li, Z., Muzikansky, A., & Ryan, D. P. (2017). Effects of early integrated palliative care in patients with lung and GI cancer: A randomized clinical trial. *Journal of Clinical Oncology, 35*(8), 834–841.

Temel, J. S., Greer, J. A., Muzikansky, A., Gallagher, E. R., Admane, S., Jackson, V. A., Dahlin, C. M., Blinderman, C. D., Jacobsen, J., Pirl, W. F., Billings, J. A., & Lynch, T. J. (2010). Early palliative care for patients with metastatic non–small-cell lung cancer. *New England Journal of Medicine, 363*(8), 733–742.

Temel, J. S., Jackson, V. A., Billings, J. A., Dahlin, C., Block, S. D., Buss, M. K., Ostler, P., Fidias, P., Muzikansky, A., Greer, J. A., Pirl, W. F., & Lynch, T. J. (2007). Phase II study: Integrated palliative care in newly diagnosed advanced non-small-cell lung cancer patients. *Journal of Clinical Oncology, 25*(17), 2377–2382.

Temel, J. S., Sloan, J., Zemla, T., Greer, J. A., Jackson, V. A., El-Jawahri, A., Kamdar, M., Kamal, A., Blinderman, C. D., Strand, J., Zylla, D., Daugherty, C., Furqan, M., Obel, J., Razaq, M., Roeland, E. J., & Loprinzi, C. (2020). Multisite, randomized trial of early integrated palliative and oncology care in patients with advanced lung and gastrointestinal cancer: Alliance A221303. *Journal of Palliative Medicine, 23*(7), 922–929.

Thomas, T. H., Jackson, V. A., Carlson, H., Rinaldi, S., Sousa, A., Hansen, A., Kamdar, M., Jacobsen, J., Park, E. R., Pirl, W. F., Temel, J. S., & Greer, J. A. (2019). Communication differences between oncologists and palliative care clinicians: A qualitative analysis of early, integrated palliative care in patients with advanced cancer. *Journal of Palliative Medicine, 22*(1), 41–49.

Thompson, L. L., Temel, B., Fuh, C. X., Server, C., Kay, P., Landay, S., Lage, D. E., Traeger, L., Scott, E., Jackson, V. A., Greer, J. A., El-Jawahri, A., Temel, J. S., & Nipp, R. D. (2020). Perceptions of medical status and treatment goal among older adults with advanced cancer. *Journal of Geriatric Oncology, 11*(6), 937–943.

Traeger, L., Rapoport, C., Wright, E., El-Jawahri, A., Greer, J. A., Park, E. R., Jackson, V. A., & Temel, J. S. (2020). Nature of discussions about systemic therapy discontinuation or hospice among patients, families, and palliative care clinicians during care for incurable cancer: A qualitative study. *Journal of Palliative Medicine, 23*(4), 542–547.

Yoong, J., Park, E. R., Greer, J. A., Jackson, V. A., Gallagher, E. R., Pirl, W. F., Back, A. L., & Temel, J. S. (2013). Early palliative care in advanced lung cancer: A qualitative study. *JAMA Internal Medicine, 173*(4), 283–290.

Adapting to the Diagnosis

A member of the palliative care team meets Alicia for the first time. They meet in the infusion bay, where the thin curtains offer symbolic privacy. Alicia is in her early 60s, and had gone to the doctor with a persistent cough. Subsequent tests revealed metastatic lung cancer. She has just finished her first cycle of first-line chemotherapy, which she tolerated well. A quick review of her chart reveals no obvious physical symptoms such as pain or shortness of breath. Her social history is notable for the recent death of her husband. She has one adult child, who lives nearby.

THE CHALLENGE OF ADAPTING TO THE DIAGNOSIS

A palliative care clinician meeting Alicia for the first time might wonder where to begin. Alicia has no obvious symptoms to address, nor is there a communication problem between the patient and the oncology team. Her disease is stable or on the way to becoming so. In this situation, a patient could be forgiven for asking, "Who are you? Why are you here?" Learning that the clinician specializes in palliative care, the patient might add, "I'm not ready for any of that stuff."

But even without the help of palliative care, Alicia has started the hard work of adapting to her diagnosis—the first challenge of serious illness. She comes to the oncology clinic for tests and infusions even though she is still in shock from the news of incurable cancer. Many patients referred for early integrated palliative care are in a similar state. Many are still adapting to a life of treatment, toxicity, recovery, and intermittent cancer monitoring. Many wonder what to expect from treatment and from the illness. Many wonder what to say to loved ones about what is happening and what might come next.

Palliative care can help patients like Alicia. Indeed, all patients with newly diagnosed serious illness face similar challenges. This first chapter discusses how palliative care clinicians can help all patients meet the first challenge of serious illness, adapting to the diagnosis. We first look at the seemingly confusing way that patients adapt to a new cancer diagnosis. Then we explore how early integrated palliative care can help. Finally, we discuss how to support our oncology colleagues starting in the early months after the patient's diagnosis.

The Beginnings of Prognostic Awareness

Receiving a diagnosis of serious illness brings the development of *prognostic awareness*: the patient's understanding of his or her most likely disease trajectory and life expectancy. At diagnosis, patients may understand only that the illness will limit their life in unspecified ways. As patients learn about their condition from their own searches, from their clinicians, or from their bodies, and with emotional support, they can develop a more accurate understanding of how much time remains and of how that time might be.

In Alicia's initial visit, she cried as she told her clinician how she had met with an attorney to draft her will. In the next moment, she talked about getting immunotherapy that might cure her cancer and was hopeful that her cancer could shrink to nothing.

A clinician could hear Alicia's talk about a possible cure as denial, as a sign that she does not understand her prognosis. The psychiatrist Dr. Avery Weisman studied hundreds of patients with cancer and observed their coping patterns. The fundamental result of his work is that denial signifies healthy coping: an effort to integrate the reality of death slowly and safely. Unlike Kübler-Ross's original schema of coping with illness, in which denial is the first of five stages of grief and acceptance the final stage, Weisman saw patients moving back and forth between denial and acceptance of impending death frequently, often within one conversation, and throughout the illness trajectory. He called this changing awareness "middle knowledge" and emphasized its coping value.

When patients get life-altering prognostic information, such as the diagnosis of metastatic cancer, they need and work to maintain emotional equilibrium. To avoid feeling overwhelmed, they titrate their illness understanding. They have worried times when they process and consider the diagnosis and hopeful times when they take a break by feeling optimistic that the disease might resolve or disappear. This patient perspective was described by Curtis et al. in a study of how patients balance hope with the desire for prognostic information: "Sometimes I feel very hopeful and think positively about the future. Other times, I feel fearful and sad because I know how serious my illness is. I seem to go back and forth between those two feelings."

We conceptualize a patient's shifting prognostic awareness as a pendulum. The pendulum swings between moments when the patient seems to understand or worry about the prognosis and moments when the patient is optimistic or hopeful about the prognosis (Figure 1.1).

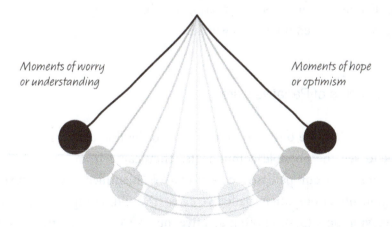

Figure 1.1 Pendulum of prognostic awareness

The pendulum encapsulates Weisman's model and reminds us that a patient's swinging awareness is healthy and normal. It describes patients' emotions as patients learn to cope with a diagnosis of serious illness, swinging to hopeful moments in order to pace the development of prognostic awareness. The pendulum model thus makes sense of a patient's contradictory expressions and reminds us that hopeful patients may have more awareness than it may seem. It helps us approach newly diagnosed patients with understanding and empathy.

Because a patient's prognostic awareness swings, it can be tricky to assess. A clinician who measures Alicia's prognostic awareness during a hopeful moment might conclude that she has not even been told that the cancer is incurable. Yet, in a realistic moment, Alicia might acknowledge the incurability and even that her life expectancy is less than a year. In Alicia's first palliative care visit, she showed both extremes.

When observing this back and forth, we don't question or correct any of the patient's statements. We just observe the swinging, know that the patient is reflecting on what he or she has been told about the illness and prognosis, and note it as a healthy response. Allowing patients to express hopes and worries without judgment builds connection that we and the patient will rely on throughout the course of the illness. Some patients may stick more to one side of the spectrum, whether being only hopeful (as discussed in Chapter 2) or being overwhelmed with worry and sadness. For all patients, this first meeting is a chance simply to observe how they swing between hopes and worries.

Components of Palliative Care

Before we describe our clinical approach to the first challenge, let's step back to see the possible components. They came from an analysis of the data from our palliative care visits. We identified seven recurring components of outpatient palliative care: (1) building rapport, (2) managing symptoms, (3) promoting adaptive coping, (4) developing prognostic awareness, (5) advance care planning, (6) facilitating treatment decisions,

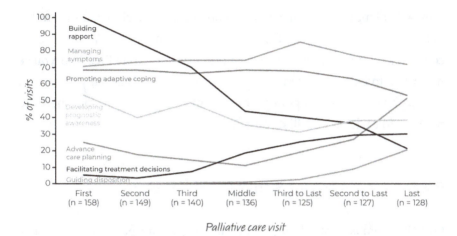

Palliative care visit

Figure 1.2 The components of palliative care across the illness trajectory

and (7) guiding disposition. Clinicians discussed most components some-time during the illness trajectory, although the timing varied (Figure 1.2). A single visit often addressed multiple components, and a component addressed in one visit might be brought up at the next or across multiple visits. In the earliest visits, the time of the first challenge, the main components are building rapport, managing symptoms, assessing prognostic awareness, and promoting adaptive coping. In the next section, we discuss how these components are combined to help patients take up this first challenge.

HOW TO HELP PATIENTS ADAPT TO THE DIAGNOSIS

In the first visits, the goal is to help patients adapt to the new diagnosis. We want our patients to get into a comfortable routine. To do that, we talk to patients about their families, jobs, or hobbies (the "building rapport" component). We also do a thorough review of symptoms and ask how they are tolerating treatment (managing symptoms). We might ask what they understand about their diagnosis or whether they have any concerns about the future (assessing prognostic awareness). We often reassure them that a cancer diagnosis is draining and that with time and support, they will adapt (promoting adaptive coping). As one clinician said to his patient, "You know what? This is completely unnerving. You've been a competent, capable person in every other area of your life. And you've never had to be a competent, capable cancer patient, but that will happen too." Applying these components may seem straightforward, but there are nuances to each, as we will discuss.

Building Rapport and the Start of Our Partnership

Our first goal is to build rapport, which begins our partnership. A critical first step is introducing the concept of palliative care to patients. Most often, the rapid pace of cancer care prevents the oncologist from introducing us and our role, so we must introduce ourselves. We used to ask patients what they knew or had been told about palliative care, but this question made them uncomfortable. Defining palliative care is often overwhelming for newly diagnosed patients. So, we now simply offer to explain the role of palliative care: "I am with the palliative care team. Would it be helpful if I gave a brief explanation of palliative care?"

For that explanation, the Center to Advance Palliative Care's definition provides a useful starting point:

> Palliative care is specialized medical care for people living with serious illness. This type of care is focused on providing relief from the symptoms and stress of a serious illness. The goal is to improve quality of life for both the patient and the family.

> Palliative care is provided by a specialty trained team of doctors, nurses, and other specialists who work together with a patient's other doctors to provide an extra layer of support. Palliative care is based on the needs of the patient, not the patient's prognosis. It is appropriate at any age and at any stage in a serious illness, and it can be provided along with curative treatment.

We generally paraphrase this definition and often emphasize our role as "quality-of-life clinicians" who will help them think ahead about important medical decisions: "I am a quality-of-life doctor. My job is to help you to live as well as possible and to be prepared for whatever lies ahead."

Occasionally we are introduced by the oncologist. Through our collaboration, oncologists have come to emphasize our role in improving quality of life and that we are part of the treatment team. One colleague uses the following language: "Palliative care is an integral part of what I do, and I cannot do what I do as well as I could without them." This support from a trusted oncologist helps wary patients trust us.

Once we have talked to the patient about the role of palliative care, we begin the symptom and psychosocial assessment. While doing our assessments, we continue to build rapport by learning about our patients' lives. Our conversations with patients about recent vacations, holiday plans, or grandchildren's graduations may look like chatting but build a connected, attuned relationship. The resulting rapport underlies our partnership with the patient. With trainee clinicians, we thus take a few minutes before we enter the room to prepare them for the rapport building in early integrated palliative care: "There will be times when the conversation feels like chatting, and you might be tempted to tune out. Don't!" We explain that conversations about the patient's life beyond the illness not only develop rapport but also serve several other important functions.

Conversations about day-to-day life cue patients that we care about more than just their experience with the cancer. We care about and enjoy who they are in the world and what is important to them. Through these conversations about day-to-day life, we see our patients more completely, and they feel known and understood by us. One clinician started this conversation by saying, "It's helpful for me to know you a little bit as a person, before all this started. Can you tell me about what you enjoy doing and a little bit about who's around you in your life?"

We may even banter about the Red Sox and the Yankees (U.S. baseball teams with a long rivalry). We show our patients that palliative care visits can be a place to laugh despite the illness. And humor builds connection.

As one clinician said to a patient, "I love when you're feeling well enough to be sarcastic, because it really makes my day to laugh."

We warn clinicians in training that these social conversations are often bidirectional. We may share details about our lives, although we do so with caution and awareness of our patient's needs. If we share too much, we draw the focus of the visit away from the patient. But our patients should feel comfortable with and connected to us. So, if our patient expresses a desire to travel to a place we know, we might mention our favorite restaurant. Or we may reveal our shared passion for baseball. Revealing a little bit of ourselves confirms that we are fellow humans, caring companions on a mysterious journey.

Assessing Symptoms Even When the Patient Feels Well

Patients early in the course of cancer often have few or even no symptoms. When we first met Alicia, just weeks after diagnosis, she had no pain and was tolerating chemotherapy. For inpatient clinicians, it can feel disorienting: How can you help a patient with few overt cancer symptoms or few treatment side effects? But we ask about symptoms anyway.

First, we often discover hidden symptoms, such as anxiety or poor sleep, that we can alleviate, whether through counseling support, lifestyle changes, or medication. As patients come to understand our role, they bring up more of their symptoms. Where they might once have considered their symptoms as "just a part of having cancer," with our help they see that symptoms can be eased or completely relieved. As one clinician said to a patient, "Don't think that you have to feel crummy just because you have cancer. Stay on us and let us know, so that we can help you feel better."

Second, identifying and alleviating symptoms builds our partnership (which will be the base for meeting the remaining challenges). One patient, Marney, could not easily adapt to functional limitations from metastases in her femur, which led to profound sorrow about her cancer. Although she could not talk about her grief, she let her palliative care clinician help with the pain. She and her clinician spoke weekly, and her clinician made small but sufficient adjustments to her medications—increasing gabapentin by 100 mg or changing the timing of the morning medications.

Building a partnership through symptom management is particularly important when patients are struggling to cope with the diagnosis. For example, sometimes an oncologist will know that a patient is struggling and reluctant to see palliative care. We suggest that the oncologist refer for management of a particular symptom, such as fatigue or insomnia. A symptom-focused referral is less threatening than a general referral. For these patients, the first palliative care visit focuses primarily or exclusively on symptom management in order to build the trust needed for harder topics. As one clinician explained, "Asking about pain or nausea is a safe topic that helps you get a full picture of where the patient is. And you can get signals of what other topics you can go into."

We begin our symptom assessment with global function: "Tell me about what a good day is like for you." This simple and patient-centered approach gives us a sense of the patient's physiological and psychological reserve. We might also learn about what is important to the patient and who is in the patient's life. We might follow up by asking about limitations: "Can you tell me more about what a tough day is like for you?" And then, "How often are you having tough days?" We fill in these global assessments with a detailed review of sleep, mood, and physical symptoms.

As a part of symptom management, we also talk with patients about what we call "scanxiety": the increased anxiety, insomnia, and irritable mood just before assessing treatment effectiveness (which is often done through CT scans but may also happen through blood work or other imaging). These symptoms are most severe when patients are newly diagnosed. We name this phenomenon for our patients so that they know what to expect and can more easily manage it. Managing scanxiety, we tell them, is a part of becoming a competent cancer patient. We also ask patients when they are due for tests, so that we can help them practice skills to manage this stressor.

Effective coping strategies to manage scanxiety include the following (which are developed in Chapter 3):

- Using a problem-solving approach by controlling the timing of tests. For example, schedule the CT scan on Monday and the follow-up visit during the week, so that patients do not have results pending over the weekend.
- Using a cognitive approach by encouraging patients to distract themselves—for example, by reading a book, planning a getaway, or doing house projects.
- Using a self-efficacy approach by reminding patients that they have the capacity to cope with whatever the scans show and that they have a team supporting them.
- Using a pharmacologic approach by prescribing intermittent medication, such as lorazepam, olanzapine, or medical marijuana.

Scanxiety rarely goes away completely. But as patients experience a few tests, they learn to anticipate and manage their symptoms. We also reassure patients that if the test results do show growth, their oncologist will work with them to determine the next best treatment. As one clinician said, "We're not going to be able to make it go away. But we hope that we give you a good, long run with the chemotherapy."

Assessing Prognostic Awareness and Tolerating Hope

Before we walk into a patient's room, we mentally draft an agenda. When patients are first adapting to the diagnosis, the agenda is modest and focuses primarily on the key components just discussed, building rapport and assessing symptoms. The rest of what we cover depends on our assessment of the patient's prognostic awareness, which, soon after diagnosis, can fluctuate rapidly.

The prognostic awareness assessment often comes with our symptom assessment. For example, we might ask about mood in an open-ended way: "How are your spirits?" The answer often offers insight into the patient's hopes and worries (the two extremes of the pendulum). If our conversation has not naturally given us a sense of our patient's prognostic awareness, we ask three questions (usually in this order):

- "What is your understanding of your illness?"
- "Looking to the future, what are your hopes for your health?"
- "What are your worries?"

If patients express wildly optimistic hopes, we know from the pendulum model that these expressions are transient and do not require recalibration or correction. In fact, patients often recalibrate their own optimistic hopes. For example, they commonly follow an optimistic hope with a more accurate expectation. One patient with refractory leukemia hoped that he would hear the words, "You're cured," caught himself, and said, "You're in remission." When patients are very hopeful, we often simply hope with them: "You are hoping for a cure. That would be so wonderful."

When the unrealistic hopes makes us uncomfortable, we think of the process of hearing, reflecting, and exploring optimistic hopes without interfering as *tolerating hope*. It is okay to tolerate hope. The possibility of dying from the cancer is too overwhelming that day. It's early in the illness trajectory, so the patient need not make any decision that day and has time to develop a more accurate understanding. Patients who receive early integrated palliative care develop more accurate prognostic awareness than patients receiving usual care.

In the pendulum model, statements of hope and worry reflect how much patients can face the illness in that moment. This capacity varies with the patient's emotional and physical state, which is why symptom management is important. Greg, a patient with metastatic pancreatic cancer, illustrated this connection for us. Early in his illness, Greg developed refractory nausea. Our appointments focused on trying medications, and Greg could talk only about how much better he hoped to feel when he was rid of the cancer. We concluded that Greg needed time to develop a more accurate understanding of his prognosis. Surprisingly, when a stent was changed in a routine procedure, his nausea abruptly resolved. With his nausea gone, Greg was able to talk at length about his worries.

Let's now look at how the three-question assessment of prognostic awareness is used to guide the rest of a conversation. The question about illness understanding probes patients' knowledge of the cancer. In contrast, the questions about hopes and worries probe how patients are adapting to that knowledge. When patients are extremely hopeful or optimistic and don't acknowledge any worries, we are cautious about inviting conversation about the future.

If we do hear a worry, we use its specificity to guide the conversation. If it's specific (for example, anxiety about an upcoming scan), we respond to the specific worry (with scanxiety, for example, offering suggestions discussed earlier in this chapter). However, a broader worry, such as, "I don't know whether I'll be able to see my daughter's wedding next year," needs a different type of conversation and a more complicated approach.

The tempting approach as a palliative care clinician is to accept the invitation to discuss prognosis. However, just after diagnosis, in-depth conversations about the prognosis often overwhelm patients, even when they seem to want to talk about the future. Rather than accepting or rejecting the invitation, we ask what kind of conversation would be most helpful. We might say, "It sounds like you are thinking about the prognosis and its impact. Part of my role is to talk about hard things like that. I know that you are newly adapting to all of this. We could talk about it more now or think about it again at a later visit. What do you think?" When we show that we can talk together about difficult topics and offer a choice in timing these discussions, patients early in the illness trajectory often choose to wait. After 1 or 2 months, we might revisit the subject: "A few visits ago, you mentioned being worried about attending your daughter's wedding. I wanted to check in with you about that."

When the patient swings from an accurate understanding back to optimistic hope, we consider ending the discussion of the future and return to tolerating hope. Patients tell us that they are starting to feel overwhelmed by redirecting the conversation toward hopes or simply changing the topic. Early in the illness trajectory, our job is to assess the patient's willingness, readiness, and ability in the moment to touch on the challenges of the illness and to follow his or her lead.

We also help the patient and family by explaining the pendulum of prognostic awareness. Patients and family members often feel confused by the patient's fluctuating hopes and worries. They feel relief when we draw the pendulum of prognostic awareness and explain that having hopeful and worried times is healthy and adaptive. One patient argued with her adult daughter because her daughter thought her too hopeful. This patient and daughter were relieved to learn that hopeful statements were healthy and not evidence of denial or an inability to face the illness.

Supporting Adaptive Coping

Just after diagnosis, patients are often overwhelmed by the diagnosis and cannot process what they've been told. To help them cope, we use the communication skills of normalizing, aligning, and containing.

NORMALIZING

We explain to patients that their emotional discomfort and upheaval are common and normal. Normalization increases patients' confidence that they will adapt to the diagnosis and early rounds of treatment. We emphasize that it is typical to feel anxious, to be unable to sleep, to be irritable, or to feel so disorganized as if the world had just exploded. We then describe a typical path through the early stages of illness, including how these feelings ease.

Here is how one clinician normalized the patient's feelings (and then offered reassurance): "What I usually say to people is, I think this time is the toughest of all because you don't know what to expect. You don't know how your body is going to feel. You don't know how the chemotherapy is going to make you feel. You don't know all the people yet. And pretty soon, you'll know everybody. They're really lovely here. And you'll know who to call for what. And that just makes it a bit easier."

ALIGNING

Next, we stress to our patients that they face the illness with our support. As one colleague said of his approach, "It's a lot of 'we.' We are going to look at this together. If anything comes up that I'm not anticipating now, we'll figure it out." So much of receiving medical care is being told what is going to happen. But when we talk with our patients about "figuring it out together," we intend a different kind of relationship, a partnership.

Alignment begins when we first meet our patients and can be that simple reassurance of figuring it out together. Then, as we help patients with symptoms, we demonstrate alignment in how we approach these concrete problems. We also show our alignment in how we help patients face the much larger existential questions of how to live with a serious illness (the theme of Chapter 3). As one clinician said, "But you guys aren't doing this alone. The first thing is, what does it mean to get diagnosed? What is the treatment going to be like? And we're going to continue to work with you to make sure you feel well in that. But the other piece is, how do you re-engage in life?"

CONTAINING

Finally, we offer permission to think less about the illness. Containment is a skill that palliative care clinicians can overlook, thinking that patients need to be doing hard emotional work. Here are several approaches for containment that emerged from our focus groups with palliative care clinicians and from our audiotaped patient encounters:

- Giving the patient permission *not* to have hard conversations. One clinician described it to us as "setting up the boundaries for these conversations. I acknowledge to patients that it's difficult to talk about their feelings about being ill. I let them know that we don't have to have that difficult conversation every day or even that day."
- Reassuring the patient that he or she will have a say in the timing of harder conversations. One clinician explained, "If the patient is pushing away and looking really anxious, I just name it. I say, 'You seem worried; what about?' And sometimes they'll say, 'That

you'll make me talk about death and dying.' And I'll say, 'I'm not going to do that. You get to guide.'"

- Providing the patient positive feedback for having engaged in hard conversations, to signal that stopping is okay. As one palliative care provider phrases it, "It seems like that was a good amount of work for today." The same provider described the role of positive feedback in containment: "Even if you wanted to accomplish two or three other things, and you just accomplished one, you make them feel good about that one because this is hard work."

- Encouraging the patient to have times to refrain from thinking about the illness. We tell our patients that it is okay to forget it all and to focus on living well and that we can have more difficult conversations when needed. As one clinician said to her patient, "I think that there are certain things that we do need to plan for, in case this doesn't go as well as what we want. And it's also really important that we try to have days when you can forget the hell about it, to the extent that you can. It's not being in denial to forget about it some days. I have to get your symptoms in good enough control so that they are not such a constant reminder."

Normalizing, aligning, and containing help patients deal with the overwhelming emotions that come with adapting to their diagnosis. But their application should not be confused with traditional psychotherapy. Although a palliative care clinician is a supportive counselor, that counseling is limited to helping the patient adapt to the illness and prognosis and thereby make informed medical decisions. For example, our role would include explaining the pendulum model to a patient and her husband so that they can better understand each other's fluctuating prognostic awareness. However, if talking about the prognosis has surfaced significant marital conflict, the patient or couple should be referred to a marital specialist. Our limited supportive counseling is not insight-oriented psychotherapy, couples or family therapy, or pediatric counseling. When needed, these services, and even intensive supportive counseling, should be offered through specialist referral.

Tips for Helping Patients Adapt to the Diagnosis

WHY

Patients experience a higher quality of life when we support their adaptation to serious illness.

WHEN

Starting at the first visit.

How

Build rapport and an aligned partnership with the patient.

Assess symptoms, even when patients feel well.

Assess prognostic awareness by asking about or listening for the patient's illness understanding, hopes, and worries.

Promote healthy coping by
- normalizing the situation: "It's normal to feel out of control in this situation. Your life has just been turned upside down. I would be worried if you weren't worried."
- aligning with the patient: "We will figure this out together."
- providing containment: "We don't have to talk about the illness."

COLLABORATING WITH COLLEAGUES

Our clinical practice follows a co-management model, meaning that palliative care and oncology clinicians together implement medical decisions. Working together includes managing the role overlap when several clinicians manage the same problem for a patient. In that situation, patients can get confused by conflicting guidance. For example, a patient might say to a palliative care clinician, "Wait, the oncologist told me to take the opioid at this dose. Why are you giving me a lower dose?" Similarly, the palliative care clinician may wonder what to say about the prognosis when the patient asks about it and reports that it has not been discussed by the oncologist. In this final section, we discuss our most important lessons about role overlap. We also discuss the palliative care clinician's unique interpretive role.

Managing Role Overlap

To understand our roles, we analyzed audio recordings of palliative care and oncology study visits, comparing the content of oncology and palliative care discussions. Although overall responsibility for care remained with the oncologist, the palliative care clinician was often responsible for key components of care such as coping support, and there were large areas of overlap between clinician's roles (Figure 1.3).

To manage role overlap, we first plan with the oncologist who will do what on a case-by-case basis. Ideally, the oncologist explicitly asks us to take charge of symptom management. Many of our oncologist colleagues often introduce us to patients naming that role: "I am going to ask palliative care to work on your pain management. They are the experts." If, however, the oncologist continues to manage basic cancer symptoms, we just explain how symptom management helps us establish rapport and trust with patients: "Would it be okay if I managed the pain? I know that

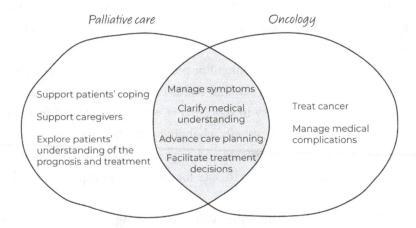

Figure 1.3 Role overlap between oncology and palliative care

you can also do it, but it is so helpful if I have something non-threatening to talk about with the patient."

Second, we manage role overlap by knowing the clinical goals. The goal may be cure, prolonged survival, better symptom control (perhaps with cancer-directed therapy), or a combination. Knowing the clinical goal and stating it clearly for the patient are particularly important when the goal is cure. We often manage symptoms in patients with curable disease such as locally advanced pancreatic cancer, head and neck cancer, or leukemia. Then we state the clinical goal of cure clearly because many patients mistakenly believe that palliative care handles only incurable illness.

Finally, as essential background, palliative care clinicians should know basic oncology, including familiarity with treatments. This shared clinical vocabulary facilitates communication and trust. It means knowing the typical first- and second-line cancer treatments and their common side effects (in common cancers with poor prognoses, including the lung and pancreas) (Box 1.1), as well as the basic milestones of progressing cancer. All this knowledge helps us to manage side effects and to help the patient understand the treatment plan and prognosis.

For example, for a patient receiving treatment for non-small-cell lung cancer, we know whether the patient is receiving standard therapy and the name of the treatment. Oncologists will at times recommend milder therapy for elderly patients or those with poor functional status, and this decision often means that the oncologist is worried that the patient may not tolerate treatment and may have a shorter prognosis. This information is critical to know.

When unsure about the treatment or prognosis, we ask the oncologist. Asking clarifies the clinical goals and builds our relationship with the oncologist. Additionally, we try to stay current with how targeted therapies and immunotherapies are rapidly changing care and prognosis. Such knowledge helps us prognosticate and set expectations for patients and families. (We often consult UpToDate for this type of rapidly changing information.)

Martha's case illustrates the value of asking. She had a rare plasmacytoma in her spine. She underwent resection followed by

---

Box 1.1 BASIC ONCOLOGY FOR PALLIATIVE CARE CLINICIANS

1. For common cancers with a poor prognosis, such as lung and pancreas:
   - Be familiar with typical first- and second-line cancer treatments and common side effects.
   - Understand the likely range of the prognosis.
   - Be aware of common presentations—for example,
     – biliary sepsis with pancreatic cancer
     – carcinomatosis with colon and other gastrointestinal cancers
     – brain metastases with small-cell lung cancer
2. For other cancers: Ask the oncologist about the prognosis and typical treatment side effects.
3. Know the cadence of treatment: Learn how many treatments are expected before the next scans and how many weeks off between treatments. (Patients can often orient you to their schedule.)
4. For targeted therapies, immunotherapy, stem cell transplant, chimeric antigen receptor (CAR)-T cells: Be familiar with them but ask questions, as they are constantly evolving.
5. Know common turning points in the illness trajectory (treatment and prognosis will vary depending on the cancer type, so we recommend discussion with the oncologist):
   - Brain metastases
   - Leptomeningeal disease
   - Pulmonary lymphangitic carcinomatosis

---

radiation with the goal of cure and was followed by palliative care for pain management. A year after treatment, she was diagnosed with multiple myeloma and came distraught to the palliative care clinic. Not fully up to date on stem cell transplantation for multiple myeloma and confused by the information on UpToDate, the palliative care clinician paged the oncologist to ask the most basic question about whether the illness was curable. It wasn't. With this information, the palliative care clinician was able to help the patient grieve and adapt. (The oncologist was relieved that the palliative care clinician called, because he had explained the prognosis to the patient but had been unsure how much she had been able to take in.)

Interpreting the Oncologist for the Patient

In focus groups with palliative care clinicians, we discovered that a key role for palliative care clinicians is being interpreters. As part of this role, we interpret the oncologist for the patient by explaining what the oncologist has said. We often begin this discussion by asking patients what they have been told: "What have you and Dr. Smith talked about related to the big picture with this cancer?" This discussion allows us to learn what the patient heard, to evaluate the patient's understanding, and to align with and maybe clarify what the oncologist said. As one colleague said, "Part of what we do is to we pick up what was said by the oncologist and feed it back to patients. We reflect it back to them in a way that they can tolerate." By explaining what the oncologist likely meant about the prognosis or treatments, we help patients develop prognostic awareness.

In the following example, the patient wants to ask about prognosis but does not do so directly. The clinician then interprets the oncologist for the patient, giving the patient a practical framework without disclosing more prognostic information than the patient can handle.

Interpreting the oncologist for the patient

PATIENT: That's another thing. What do—all right, I go through this treatment. Say the prognosis reduces again. What's the long-term effect of the prognosis on this thing? How long can this thing go? What happens? No one knows?

PALLIATIVE CARE CLINICIAN: It's hard to know for sure. We look at how you're doing using the scans. If the chemotherapy is continuing to work, he'll keep you on that. Some people live years with this. They can. It's really unusual, but there are people who have. They have cancer that's a little bit stupid and cannot outsmart the chemotherapy, right? (laughter) The chemotherapy easily keeps it in check. Now, I hope that you're one of the guys who's got cancer like that. And we'll see. Scans will give us information. So, if we see that the scan looks good, he'll stay the course. If it looks like it's growing, and he doesn't think this chemotherapy is working, then he'll switch you to something else.

PATIENT: Okay.

Interpreting the Patient for the Oncologist

The other direction of our interpreter role is interpreting the patient for the oncologist, often explaining what the patient understands about the prognosis. Patients often struggle to take in prognostic information, even when it is clearly explained, particularly early in the course of the illness. As illustrated by the pendulum, patients integrate prognostic information at a pace that preserves their ability to function in the world. So, they might not at first remember or report back information that is too overwhelming. For example, patients will frequently talk about getting rid of the cancer, beating the cancer, or getting the cancer out of their body, even when the oncologist has described the incurable prognosis clearly. Interpreting the patient, we reassure the oncologist that the patient's lack of understanding does not mean that the oncologist was not skilled in communicating (and we might offer the pendulum model by way of explanation).

We also interpret the patient for the oncologist by identifying patients who are struggling. As one clinician put it, "I will say to the oncologist, 'I am a little concerned about what [the patient] is understanding.'" In such cases, the patient and family may need additional clarification from the oncologist. For example, the oncologist might have to confirm gently that the goal of treatment is not cure. We see this need occasionally in patients with glioblastomas. The patient hears from the surgeon that they "got it all" and from the radiation oncologist that that the treatment went well, and the patient comes to our clinic not understanding that the tumor is incurable and the likely prognosis is less than a year.

In addition to interpreting the patient's prognostic awareness, we also share important information about the patient's priorities. As one palliative care clinician noted, "There are things patients will tell us in palliative care visits that they won't tell the oncologist, not because they don't care about the oncologist but because they worry that they're going to let the oncologist down or that the oncologist won't see them anymore if they don't want more chemotherapy." In one case, our highlighting a patient's neuropathy helped the oncologist choose a chemotherapy. The patient, a pianist, had not wanted to emphasize his neuropathy symptoms, fearing that he would get less potent chemotherapy. In truth, the chemotherapy options had equal potential. When the oncologist understood the degree of neuropathy and its effect on the patient's piano playing, he chose a regimen that carried less risk of neuropathy.

Sometimes our interpreter role means encouraging patients to communicate more of their thinking with the oncologist. For example, after helping our patient choose priorities, we encourage the patient to talk with the oncologist or suggest a joint visit. Or, we get permission from the patient to share the relevant parts of the discussion with the oncologist.

Although interpreting occurs in inpatient palliative care, the role is more developed in early integrated palliative care. Long-term relationships with patients and oncologists foster a more nuanced understanding of how each party thinks, making us more effective interpreters.

Joint Visits

The most direct form of interpretation occurs when we spend time together in same room with the oncologist and the patient in a joint visit. We interpret the oncologist and the patient best when we hear directly what they say to each other. We can pick up subtle emotional cues or probe when the patient does not seem to understand the prognostic information that the oncologist is sharing. We can also help the patient work through strong emotions, making the oncologist less tempted to offer treatments because the patient is desperate or overwhelmed. As an oncology colleague told us, "It helps to have you in the room with me so that I stick with my plan. I don't want to offer things in the moment that I don't really think will help. But it is just so hard to respond to desperation when I am alone."

Oncologists also appreciate joint visits for increasing their skill and knowledge of palliative care. Oncologists who are more comfortable talking about prognosis, advance care planning, and death and dying have higher rates of generalist palliative care delivery and specialist palliative care referral. Joint visits have helped build our collaborative practice.

Finally, patients also welcome joint visits. They appreciate coordinated care, particularly at a transition, such as when reviewing a scan result or making a new treatment plan. Patients then feel overwhelmed and need visibly organized support from the medical team. Having both clinicians in the room efficiently signals to the patient and family that the team is in agreement on considering next steps.

Here is an example from a joint visit. The oncologist has decided to stop chemotherapy in order to offer radiation for an acute bleed, but the patient fears stopping chemotherapy.

Aligning with the oncologist's plan

PATIENT: So, I mean, what happens with the chemotherapy?

ONCOLOGIST: I want to get to the plan. The plan is to get radiation.

PALLIATIVE CARE CLINICIAN: And that's our hope, too, that the radiation helps stop this bleeding, and we can get back to chemotherapy. That's the plan.

PATIENT: Right.

PALLIATIVE CARE CLINICIAN: The other thing that has been hard about this, and there have been so many hard things, is that there hasn't been any time to have a breather, to get out of the weeds and think. It just feels like it has been one crisis after another. And what I want— what my hope is for you, is that we just get some time with no drama.

PATIENT: No drama.

ONCOLOGIST: In general, it is easier for patients and families to think about long-term plans during periods of no drama. Right now, it's hard for all of us to think long term when we just want to get through this.

In this joint visit, the palliative care clinician reiterates the oncologist's plan, and the oncologist reiterates the palliative care clinician's hopes for a time without drama. This echoing demonstrates mutual respect and that the clinicians are aligned.

MEETING THE CHALLENGE OF ADAPTING TO THE DIAGNOSIS

In this chapter, we discussed how to work with patients soon after diagnosis to help them adapt. Adaptation is ongoing. However, patients have substantially met this first challenge once their symptoms are under control and they have established a treatment routine: managing visits (including palliative care), labs, scans, treatment, symptoms, medications, and side effects. Then patients will have the cognitive and emotional reserve to consider the second challenge, pairing hopes and worries.

COMMUNICATION SKILLS SUMMARY

CHAPTER 1: ADAPTING TO THE DIAGNOSIS

Assess prognostic awareness: What is your understanding of your illness? Looking to the future, what are your hopes? What are your worries?

Support coping: Normalize the patient's experience, align with the patient, and contain the patient's overwhelming emotions.

Be an interpreter: Interpret the patient for the oncologist and the oncologist for the patient.

FURTHER READING

Bakitas, M., Lyons, K. D., Hegel, M. T., & Ahles, T. (2013). Oncologists' perspectives on concurrent palliative care in a National Cancer Institute-designated comprehensive cancer center. *Palliative and Supportive Care, 11*(5), 415–423.

Center to Advance Palliative Care. (2011). *Public opinion research on palliative care: A report based on research by Public Opinion Strategies.* https://www.capc.org/Curtis, J. R., Engelberg, R., Young, J. P., Vig, L. K., Reinke, L. F., Wenrich, M. D., McGrath, B., McCown, E., & Back, A. L. (2008). An approach to understanding the interaction of hope and desire for explicit prognostic information among individuals with severe chronic obstructive pulmonary disease or advanced cancer. *Journal of Palliative Medicine, 11*(4), 610–620.

Fujisawa, D., Temel, J. S., Traeger, L., Greer, J. A., Lennes, I. T., Mimura, M., & Pirl, W. F. (2015). Psychological factors at early stage of treatment as predictors of receiving chemotherapy at the end of life. *Psycho-Oncology, 24*(12), 1731–1737.

Hannon, B., O'Reilly, V., Bennett, K., Breen, K., & Lawlor, P. (2012). Meeting the family: Measuring effectiveness of family meetings in a specialist inpatient palliative care unit. *Palliative and Supportive Care, 10*(1), 43–49.

Hudson, P., Thomas, T., Quinn, K., & Aranda, S. (2009). Family meetings in palliative care: Are they effective? *Palliative Medicine, 23*(2), 150–157.

Jackson, V. A., Jacobsen, J., Greer, J. A., Pirl, W. F., Temel, J. S., & Back, A. L. (2013). The cultivation of prognostic awareness through the provision of early palliative care in the ambulatory setting: A communication guide. *Journal of Palliative Medicine, 16*(8), 894–900.

Jacobs, J. M., Shaffer, K. M., Nipp, R. D., Fishbein, J. N., MacDonald, J., El-Jawahri, A., Pirl, W. F., Jackson, V. A., Park, E. R., Temel, J. S., & Greer, J. A. (2017). Distress is interdependent in patients and caregivers with newly diagnosed incurable cancers. *Annals of Behavioral Medicine, 51*(4), 519–531.

Jacobsen, J., Thomas, J. D., & Jackson, V. A. (2013). Misunderstandings about prognosis: An approach for palliative care consultants when the patient does not seem to understand what was said. *Journal of Palliative Medicine, 16*(1), 91–95.

Kübler-Ross, E. (1969). *On death and dying.* Macmillan.

Nipp, R. D., El-Jawahri, A., Fishbein, J. N., Gallagher, E. R., Stagl, J. M., Park, E. R., Jackson, V. A., Pirl, W. F., Greer, J. A., & Temel, J. S. (2016). Factors associated with depression and anxiety symptoms in family caregivers of patients with incurable cancer. *Annals of Oncology, 27*(8), 1607–1612.

Paladino, J., Lakin, J. R., & Sanders, J. J. (2019). Communication strategies for sharing prognostic information with patients: Beyond survival statistics. *Journal of the American Medical Association* [online ahead of print].

Temel, J. S., Greer, J. A., Admane, S., Gallagher, E. R., Jackson, V. A., Lynch, T. J., Lennes, I. T., Dahlin, C. M., & Pirl, W. F. (2011). Longitudinal perceptions of prognosis and goals of therapy in patients with metastatic non-small-cell lung cancer: Results of a randomized study of early palliative care. *Journal of Clinical Oncology, 29*(17), 2319–2326.

Temel, J. S., Jackson, V. A., Billings, J. A, Dahlin, C., Block, S. D., Buss, M. K., Ostler, P., Fidias, P., Muzikansky, A., Greer, J. A., Pirl, W. F., & Lynch T. J. (2007). Phase II study: Integrated palliative care in newly diagnosed advanced non-small-cell lung cancer patients. *Journal of Clinical Oncology, 25*(17), 2377–2382.

Temel, J. S., McCannon, J., Greer, J. A., Jackson, A., Ostler, P., Pirl, W. F., Lynch, T. J., & Billings, J. A. (2008). Aggressiveness of care in a prospective cohort of patients with advanced NSCLC. *Cancer, 113*(4), 826–833.

Thomas, T. H., Jackson, V. A., Carlson, H., Rinaldi, S., Sousa, A., Hansen, A., Kamdar, M., Jacobsen, J., Park, E. R., Pirl, W. F., Temel, J. S., & Greer, J. A. (2019). Communication differences between oncologists and palliative care clinicians: A qualitative analysis of early, integrated palliative care in patients with advanced cancer. *Journal of Palliative Medicine, 22*(1), 41–49.

Weisman, A. (1972). *On dying and denying.* Behavioral Publications, Inc.

Weisman, A. D., & Worden, J. W. (1976). The existential plight in cancer: Significance of the first 100 days. *International Journal of Psychiatry in Medicine, 7*(1), 1–15.

Yoong, J., Park, E. R., Greer, J. A., Jackson, V. A., Gallagher, E. R., Pirl, W. F., Back, A. L., & Temel, J. S. (2013). Early palliative care in advanced lung cancer: A qualitative study. *JAMA Internal Medicine, 173*(4), 283–290.

Pairing Hopes and Worries

George, an engineer recently diagnosed with incurable pancreatic cancer, was making his first palliative care visit. He was warm and welcoming but had not heard of palliative care. Asked by his palliative care clinician about his hopes, he said that he was 100% focused on beating the cancer. Over several visits, he described in detail his new interest in medical science. Since his diagnosis, he had been reading cancer journals with a particular interest in breakthroughs in immunotherapy and targeted therapy. He talked a lot about how these new therapies might be applied to pancreatic cancer. Asked about his worries, George replied that he had none.

THE CHALLENGE OF PAIRING HOPES AND WORRIES

A clinician working with George might feel stuck. George has given clear cues that he will not talk about or consider the possibility of dying from the cancer. The clinician would want to respect George's cues and build trust and rapport. If pushed too hard, George might fire the clinician. That same clinician would also know that George would benefit from thinking about the future of his illness, so that he can begin to adapt to its most likely course.

Whereas the previous chapter described the importance of supporting a patient's hopes, even hopes that are unrealistically optimistic, this chapter focuses on the second challenge: pairing hopes with worries (Figure 2.1).

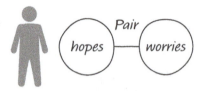

Figure 2.1 Challenge 2: pairing hopes and worries

Meeting this challenge is important because patients who cannot face worries will remain unrealistically optimistic about their prognosis even when approaching end of life. Over time, the growing divide between the patient's unrealistic expectations and the clinical reality distresses the entire medical team and pulls everyone—patient, medical team, and caregivers—toward aggressive care at end of life, care that is unlikely to extend or improve life and is likely to cause suffering.

In this chapter, we first describe how difficult it is for anyone to acknowledge mortality. We then explain how, by pairing hopes and worries, patients develop a broader perspective on the illness that promotes quality of life and preparation for end of life. Next we describe communication skills for helping patients pair hopes and worries. Finally, we offer suggestions for talking with oncology colleagues about a patient's developing prognostic awareness.

THE THREAT OF MORTALITY

A diagnosis of serious illness awakens patients to their mortality and evokes thoughts and feelings that are difficult even to consider. Indeed, emerging neuroscience research points to an ancient mechanism that shields us from this existential fear: Our brain resists linking the self with death and categorizes death as an event that exclusively befalls others. Long ago, this defense was probably balanced by the ubiquity of death. But with declining mortality rates and with the dying sequestered to hospitals, hospices, and nursing homes, we are less exposed to dying and therefore less psychologically prepared for end of life. Thus, the struggle to acknowledge the possibility of dying reflects a normal, perhaps ancient, psychological tendency reinforced by the wider culture.

This struggle is represented in the pendulum introduced in Chapter 1 (Figure 1.1), which illustrates that many patients consider mortality only briefly before counterbalancing these worrying thoughts with a swing to hopes. Some patients, like George, may hear the diagnosis, become deeply worried, swing to hopes, and stay there, where they focus on optimistic, often unrealistic hopes. We describe these patients as having *low prognostic awareness*.

A psychologically informed palliative care clinician caring for George would not get frustrated or stuck by his optimism. Rather, the clinician would recognize that George has worries that he is suppressing. Taking in such intense fears and worries may be too distressing all at once. Thus, the clinician would slowly develop a partnership, building rapport and managing symptoms while exploring worries safely, pacing conversations about worries according to George's ability to cope and the clinical urgency.

CLINICAL ATTUNEMENT

Helping patients begin the emotionally challenging process of acknowledging worries requires *attunement*. Attunement is a term from the attachment literature that describes an awareness of and responsiveness to another's situation, in which both people feel a resonance or synchrony. Attunement extends beyond empathy, which is simply being aware of and responsive to another's feelings. To empathy, attunement adds responsiveness to other needs, including needs for information, medical care, privacy, or autonomy.

Attunement requires clinicians to shift their own internal state, awareness, and actions to understand the inner world and needs of the patient. It is expressed through the clinician's words and actions, including nonverbal actions. Consider symptom management. As a clinician responds to a patient's symptoms, assessing and managing them, the clinician understands the symptoms, and senses the patient's personality, mood, ability to cope with and manage problems, and perhaps the patient's place within a family system. Furthermore, this understanding is bidirectional: The patient recognizes the clinician as a person who can empathize with and respond to his or her needs. When the clinician's response matches the needs of the patient, the patient feels known and understood and therefore less alone with the illness.

For example, a clinician hears a patient say, "My pain is fine," but knows that this patient tends to underreport symptoms. By asking further, the clinician demonstrates attunement. An attuned clinician might also know whether a patient who brings an adult child to the visit wants a deeper discussion about the future to inform the family member or whether the visitor signals that the patient prefers to keep things positive. Furthermore, an attuned clinician who did not know would ask, "It is lovely to meet your daughter. Can you give me a sense of what would be most important for us to cover today?"

To specialize the concept of attunement, which is critical in psychologically therapeutic relationships, we introduce the term *clinical attunement*. This term includes the aspects of attunement specific to palliative care: being aware of and responsive to the patient's hopes and worries and understanding the most likely timeframe and illness trajectory.

WHY PAIRING HOPES AND WORRIES IS IMPORTANT

Some patients, such as George, seem focused solely on hope. Others seem overwhelmed and focus solely on worries. Many patients, such as Alicia (from Chapter 1), alternate between hopes and worries. All of these patients, represented in Figure 2.2a, have not (yet) paired hopes and worries.

This pairing can seem like such a small thing. Why bother? But pairing hopes and worries, understanding that these opposite feelings can occur together, improves patients' experience of illness. Because hopes and worries are not easily reconciled opposites, pairing them requires a certain emotional and cognitive distance (Figure 2.2b). Patients need to

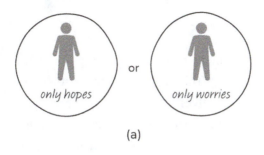

(a)

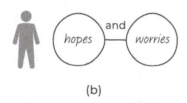

(b)

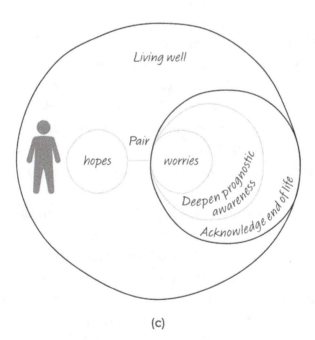

(c)

Figure 2.2 Hopes and worries integrated into a unified perspective over time
(a) Where the patient started. Around diagnosis, the patient is surrounded by either hopes or worries.
(b) The awareness the patient reaches in this challenge. To pair hopes and worries, which are opposites, a certain distance is required.
(c) Where the five challenges take the patient: the integrated self. Once paired, hopes and worries can inform each other and expand to the more complex goals of living well and acknowledging end of life, discussed in Chapters 3, 4, and 5.

step outside their moment-to-moment feelings enough to see hopes and worries simultaneously. This slight distance, with its fuller perspective, helps patients see themselves with clarity and empathy.

Pairing of hopes and worries builds the foundation for meeting the subsequent challenges. A hopeful perspective tempered by worries can be expanded beyond cure or prolonging survival to the idea of living well (Figure 2.2c), which also includes other hopes such as feeling better or having quality time with loved ones. (The challenge of living well is discussed in Chapter 3.) Similarly, a worried perspective buoyed by hope can be expanded beyond inchoate fears to a more nuanced acknowledgment of dying (discussed in Chapters 4 and 5). As each perspective expands and becomes more nuanced, it strengthens the other. The expansion and mutual strengthening of hopes and worries leads to their integration and develops the patient's integrated self: a unified perspective of living well while acknowledging end of life.

We often see patients develop the integrated self. Terry, a man in his early 50s with sarcoma, hoped to control his cancer for a long time and acknowledged that his illness prevented him from working or traveling. Yet he didn't want to talk about any worries. He used distraction to avoid overwhelming thoughts, filling his time watching nature webcams. He was engrossed specifically with watching the birth and growth of a baby giraffe.

Over time, Terry's clinician invited him to talk more about worries gently paired with hopes. In accepting the invitation, Terry, though terrified of the future, acknowledged his mortality. In turn, this acknowledgment deepened his appreciation of the giraffe. The giraffe reminded him of the cycle of life and offered him hope for the continuity of life beyond his own. In his remaining time, Terry raised awareness of and money for endangered wildlife. By acknowledging worries, Terry lived more fully.

Importantly, although integrating hopes and worries is the goal of our clinical work, patients need not maintain this perspective continuously. They can still have solely hopeful times. These times give patients a break from thinking about the illness. Conversely, they can also have deeply sad and worried times. These times enable grieving and planning. Patients will still swing on the pendulum.

HOW TO HELP PATIENTS PAIR HOPES AND WORRIES

We first describe our pairing approach for patients like George, who have low prognostic awareness and focus solely on hopes. We then discuss how to help patients like Alicia, who alternate between hopes and worries and need only gentle guidance to pair them. Some patients pair hopes and worries on their own by using "hope for the best and prepare for the worst." When we help patients with this challenge, however, we prefer the "hopes and worries" pairing as less extreme and more integrated, allowing for more realistic hopes and worries that are less frightening.

Patients Focused Solely on Hope

What if a patient expresses no concerns about the future and insists on staying optimistic? Fortunately, just having a palliative care clinician in the room helps these patients acknowledge worries, even if they feel well and we talk only about their upcoming vacation. Once patients understand the meaning of palliative care and tolerate our presence, they have implicitly acknowledged a serious illness and we can begin to work with them on pairing hopes and worries.

SKILLS FOR PAIRING HOPES AND WORRIES

We first align and thereby validate patients' hopes. We do so by echoing patients' hopes using their words. For example, when George says that he is 100% focused on beating the cancer, we repeat back: "I know that you are 100% focused on beating this cancer." Then, we introduce worries. We do so by touching upon the illness gently. (This pairing could happen anytime during the visit.) Here are several ways. In each example, the

Table 2.1 WAYS TO TOUCH UPON THE ILLNESS GENTLY

Empathizing	Empathize with the experience of the illness. **"I know you are 100% focused on beating the cancer.** *It is hard to live with the uncertainty of a serious illness."*
Understanding the illness's impact on others	Ask about how family or friends are coping. **"I know you are 100% focused on beating this cancer.** *How is your family doing with all of this?"*
Suggesting a worried part	Suggest that a part of the patient may be worried. **"I know you are 100% focused on beating the cancer.** *I imagine there is also a part of you that worries about what might lie ahead."*
Mentioning the "what ifs"	Use the "what ifs" to hold the possibility of dying at a safer distance. **"I know you are 100% focused on beating the cancer.** *Part of my job is to invite you to think ahead and prepare for the 'what ifs'."*
Linking to worries with "even though"	Use "even though" to link a reframed hope to the illness. **"I know you are 100% focused on beating the cancer. Our challenge together is to help you live well** *even though we are facing this illness."*

alignment with hope is bolded and the touch upon the illness is italicized (Table 2.1).

Empathizing

We imagine what the patient is going through and give words to our thoughts.

- **"I know that you are 100% focused on beating this cancer.** *It is hard to live with the uncertainty of a serious illness."*
- **"I know you are 100% focused on beating this cancer.** *It is so difficult even to have to think about all of this."*
- **"I know you are 100% focused on beating this cancer.** *You have been through a lot with this diagnosis."*

Statements of empathy gently acknowledge what patients are going through without asking them to talk more about what is to come.

Understanding the Illness's Impact on Others

Asking about the impact of the illness on family or friends invites patients to acknowledge worries indirectly.

- **"I know you are 100% focused on beating this cancer.** *How is your family doing with all of this?"*

Often a patient will say only that a loved one is worried, but even this response indirectly acknowledges the patient's worries.

Suggesting a Worried Part

This construct suggests that just a part of the patient may be worried.

- **"I know that you are 100% focused on beating this cancer.** *I imagine there is also a part of you that worries about what might lie ahead. "*

The "parts" concept has been developed extensively in internal family systems (IFS) therapy. It is useful because, even when patients at first reject the seriousness of the illness, they can often hear it softly by acknowledging a worried part. (The preceding example dialog also adds the hypothetical framing: "I imagine . . .")

In our experience, most patients can acknowledge a worried part, often simply by nodding. We then recognize this emotional accomplishment and empathize: "This is such a hard situation that you are facing." With very hopeful patients, simply making this acknowledgment may be enough progress for one visit. We then suggest a later conversation: "Maybe next time we can talk more about the part of you that worries."

For a few patients, even acknowledging a worried part is too distressing. These patients instead redirect the conversation back to hopes: "Right now I just want to stay positive." In such cases, we align: "I hear that it is very important to stay positive. Let's focus on what we can do to help you feel your best." We will try again with this or another pairing approach at future visits.

Mentioning the "what ifs."

The "what ifs" hold the possibility of dying at a safer (subjunctive) distance.

- **"I know you are 100% focused on beating this cancer.** *Part of what I do is to think ahead and help you prepare for the 'what ifs'."*

This construct incorporates doubt about what might happen, suggesting that something unwanted *could* rather than will happen. We then see how patients respond. When patients make eye contact or nod, we know that they can tolerate our indirect reference to end of life. When patients are uncomfortable with it, they often suggest a different focus for our visits: "I think my oncologist wanted you to help with my pain." We then focus on the patient's pain and other symptoms for the remainder of the visit. We might spend several visits focusing on symptoms and coping (as detailed in Chapter 3) before again pairing hopes and worries.

Linking with "even though."

The "even though" conjunction can link the illness to a reframed hope.

- **"I hear that you are 100% focused on beating this cancer. Our challenge together is to figure out how to help you live well** *even though we are facing this illness."*

In this example, the clinician aligns with the patient's hope and then names an additional hope, to live well. The "even though" construct is a stronger touch upon the illness because it implies the illness's continued presence. Thus, to avoid a jarring transition, before pairing, the clinician first reframes the patient's hope to a more achievable goal (living well).

The following example illustrates these approaches with George. He is still focused on a scientific breakthrough that will bring a cure. By repeatedly aligning with George's hopes, the clinician shows George that she understands the importance to him of hope. After each alignment, the clinician touches upon the illness.

Touching upon the illness

Dialog	Our perspective
CLINICIAN: George, I know that it is very important for you that we stay positive and focus on how science might help you beat this illness. It is difficult even to have to think about all of this.	*Aligns with George's hope and empathizes with the illness experience.*
GEORGE: Yes, it is important for me to keep a positive attitude. I want to meet my grandchildren!	*Stresses the importance of optimism.*
CLINICIAN: Yes, it is very important to keep a positive attitude. Part of my role is to help patients find ways to live well even though we are facing illness.	*Aligns with hope and living well, and touches upon the illness with "even though."*
GEORGE: Well, right now, my life is focused on beating this cancer. I think that immunotherapy could enable my body to heal.	*Redirects the conversation to his hopes.*
CLINICIAN: Absolutely, living your life and deciding how to fight this cancer are important. Sometimes patients also have a part of them that worries. Our visits can be a place where we can talk about both, if or when that is helpful.	*Aligns with hope and suggests that George might have a worried part and that this clinical relationship is a safe place to explore worries.*
GEORGE: Well, I do worry, but I don't want to be negative. I will think about it. I am glad that you are here to help.	*Has heard the pairing and expresses gratitude for the relationship.*
CLINICIAN: This is a tough situation.	*Empathizes.*

When we first pair hopes and worries, we watch and listen for any readiness to talk further about worries. Patients may simply nod or agree. We might make a pairing several times, as the above example illustrates, touching upon the illness in several ways or in one way several times before the patient acknowledges any concerns.

MODERATE DIFFICULTY

It might seem unattuned or unaligned to keep touching upon the illness when patients indicate that they want to be hopeful. However, with the illness inevitably come worries. We don't create them by talking about them. Rather, when patients can safely talk about them, they feel seen, supported, and relieved. For example, oncology patients show a sustained reduction in anxiety after a serious illness conversation. As Mister Rogers, the famous children's television host, says, "What is mentionable is manageable."

Once George says, "I do worry," he has heard the pairing and feels safe enough to acknowledge worried feelings within the clinical relationship. Then it is safe for the clinician to touch again upon the illness, which she does by expressing empathy, and to acknowledge and perhaps to explore George's worries at a future visit.

When helping patients pair hopes and worries so that they eventually integrate these contrasting perspectives, we do not rush. In early integrated palliative care, patients have time. Understanding the medical context and knowing how much a patient can think about the future, we offer them a conversation of moderate difficulty. This level of challenge helps patients learn to integrate hopes and worries without feeling overwhelmed.

Presenting a moderate difficulty[1] helped one author's child learn to swim. Her daughter had been paddling around every evening in a swim vest for months without learning to swim. In frustration, her husband purchased a second swim vest with six removable Styrofoam floaters. Each evening he removed one floater, giving the daughter a moderate difficulty. After four floaters had been removed, she said, "Take off the vest" and

---

1. In education research, this idea is known as the principle of moderate challenge.

could swim. Four evenings of moderate difficulty achieved what months of insufficient difficulty could not.

The principle of moderate difficulty offers the clinician a route between two common and contrasting pitfalls in palliative care: leading the patient into emotional chaos or leaving the patient rigidly hopeful. (This schema of steering a course between chaos and rigidity is discussed by Daniel Siegel and Tina Bryson.) The chaos pitfall happens when we don't pay enough attention to patients' distress. Rushing patients to explore worries in depth (taking off the swim vest all at once), we either get fired or break trust, which complicates further exploration. The rigidity pitfall happens when we pay too much attention to patients' distress, seeing exclusive expressions of hope as barring exploration of worries. Assuming that patients focused only on hope cannot pair and eventually integrate hopes and worries, we never touch upon the illness (we never remove a floater). But without that moderate difficulty, these patients remain unrealistically hopeful. Fortunately, by touching upon the illness gently, and with the grace of time, patients will usually pair hopes and worries.

That's what happened with George. Although he did not specify his worries, he confirmed their existence, which had an important effect. A few weeks later, George took early retirement, even though he remained focused on scientific breakthroughs. When we asked him about his decision, George said that he had been thinking more about his cancer. He seemed to have a deeper sense of the prognosis, saying, "I don't know what lies ahead. But I figure I may as well enjoy myself. I've got a whole lot saved up. I want to make sure I spend it well."

Integrating the Approach into Clinical Practice

In summary, for patients who express only hopes, we use their words to align with their hopes and then gently explore their ability to acknowledge worries in a way that is empathic and attuned.

Figure 2.3 shows how clinicians can apply this approach. As illustrated with George, we often present the pairing several times, even over several visits. Pairing is a gentle invitation to difficult work. We are mindful to recognize even small steps, such as a patient's worried statement or expression. Because patients in early integrated palliative care are usually clinically

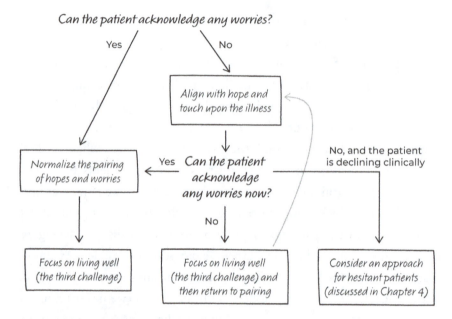

Figure 2.3 Integrating the approach into clinical practice

stable, they have time to go slowly. Over several months, as we build rapport and address symptoms, we look for opportunities to retest their tolerance for pairing. Once patients acknowledge worries, we normalize the pairing of hope and worries, which is discussed in the next section.

A few patients refuse our invitations to acknowledge worries. These patients may cancel visits or object to any focus other than symptom management. With these patients, we skip to the third challenge, living well with serious illness (Chapter 3). Patients will then learn coping skills that help them acknowledge worries, and we can again invite them to pair hopes and worries. (Occasionally, when patients are very hesitant to ac-knowledge worries despite these efforts and are declining clinically, we skip to the specialist approach discussed in Chapter 4.)

Patients Who Can Acknowledge Hopes and Worries

Some patients (like Alicia) express fluctuating hopes or worries. For ex-ample, in one moment Alicia hopes immunotherapy might melt her cancer away to nothing; in the next, she talks about drafting her will. We help these patients to pair their hopes and worries, normalizing that these contrasting feelings can coexist.

When patients can acknowledge hopes and worries, the pairing is straightforward. We just echo to the patient the hopes and worries expressed during the visit and normalize that mixed feelings about the future are healthy and helpful. To Alicia, we might say, "I hear you are hoping that the treatment can help and possibly even lead to a sustained remission, and you are worried enough to draft a will and prepare your estate. Being hopeful and worried is a healthy way of coping."

In the audiotaped example below, the clinician explores and pairs the patient's hopes and worries.

Pairing already present hopes and worries

Dialog	Our perspective
CLINICIAN: How are you making sense of the illness, in terms of your understanding of what to expect?	*Invites a conversation about worries.*
PATIENT: So I believe, I know it's going to work out, and I know my lifespan's going to be extended, and I can already feel the changes in my body.	
CLINICIAN: So you're hopeful that the treatment can help.	*Aligns with hope.*
PATIENT: But I'm still a very pragmatic individual, and I know the percentages.	
CLINICIAN: Right. So you feel that, even if you do well with this, this is likely what you'll die from.	*Names the worry explicitly in a way that the patient could not.*

Dialog	Our perspective
Patient: Oh, yeah. I'm pretty sure. I have to be realistic, I have to be true to myself, and that's what bothers me.	*Confirms that it is okay for the clinician to be explicit about dying.*
Clinician: Because it's how to live in both worlds?	*Pairs hopes and worries, framed as a question to allow the patient to endorse or reject this perspective.*
Patient: Yeah.	*Endorses the pairing.*

In this example, the clinician interprets the patient's experience for the patient—a crucial skill discussed here and in Chapter 4. The clinician invites a conversation about the future and reflects back what the patient says while synthesizing and clarifying the patient's implicit meaning. Interpreting the patient for the patient has several benefits. First, it gives patients language for emotions hard to describe and thoughts hard to articulate, helping them face topics difficult to confront. Second, it shows them that they can tolerate these discussions and need not be overwhelmed. Finally, it helps the clinician reflect back hopes and worries as pairs (often within a sentence). Once a patient understands healthy coping includes hopes and worries and can assent to their pairing, the patient has met the second challenge of serious illness.

Tips for Helping Patients Pair Hopes and Worries

WHY

Pairing hopes and worries shows patients that having a range of thoughts and feelings about the illness is healthy and prepares them to take up the remaining challenges.

WHEN

Begin once patients have met the first challenge: Their symptoms are managed and they are comfortable with their new cancer routine.

How

Pair hopes and worries based on the patient's ability to acknowledge worries.

For patients who focus solely on hope. Align with hope and touch upon the illness by

- empathizing: "My job is to help you live well. *It is hard to live with the uncertainty of cancer.*"
- understanding the illness's impact on others: "*How is your family doing with all of this?*"
- suggesting a worried part: "I know that your goal is to be positive and to live well. I imagine that there is also *a part of you that worries.*"
- mentioning the "what ifs": "A big part of my job is helping you to live well; another part is to talk with you to think ahead and prepare for *the what ifs.*"
- linking to worries with "even though": "My job is to help you live well *even though* we are facing this illness."

For patients who acknowledge hopes and worries. Pair the patient's hopes and worries, and then normalize the mixed feelings.

COLLABORATING WITH COLLEAGUES

With the oncologist, we don't talk about the specialist details of pairing. Instead, we refer to the pendulum (Figure 1.1), a model for the oncologist to interpret the patient. We might say, "George is starting to swing on the pendulum. As you know, he has been very hopeful. In my last conversation, he did acknowledge that a part of him worries. He is glad that we are involved. I think that I will be able to help him talk more about the hard stuff."

Many of our colleagues know the pendulum model as we have been teaching it at our institution for years. With new clinicians, the model is quick to explain. "In palliative care, we have noticed that patients cope with illness by having hopeful times and worried times. We think of this back and forth as a pendulum. It's a healthy way to cope."

Through our collaboration, our colleagues have learned that patients will eventually take in prognostic information, even if they cannot seem to at first. They have also learned that, early in the illness, there is no hurry. Even optimistic patients will understand the prognosis with time and palliative care support. One colleague described his own process for understanding how patients develop prognostic awareness:

> I used to be somebody who needed to get the patient onto my wavelength, in terms of the cancer, as fast as I could. And I probably came across a little bit like somebody with a baseball bat just hammering away, "No. You have to think this way about the cancer. And this is your prognosis." What I learned from the palliative care physicians is that prognostic awareness is a series of understandings and that not everybody has to get onto the same page all at once.

For our oncology colleagues, we also identify patients who struggle to pair hopes and worries. When we describe these patients' prognostic awareness to the oncologist, we often find that the oncologist is also worried. These patients give confusing signals about what they understand, but several patterns are common.

The first pattern is exemplified by George, whose pendulum of prognostic awareness remains fixed at the optimistic side. We tell our oncology colleagues that this one-sided thinking is normal early in the disease trajectory and often eases with time or as we help the patient pair hopes and worries (as described in this chapter). But for patients stuck in this pattern, we recommend close palliative care follow-up and use the approach for patients who are hesitant described in Chapter 4.

In the second pattern, patients are fixed at hopeless realism. These patients talk about the illness and prognosis, often sharing detailed plans for end of life, but have difficulty pairing their often accurate understanding of the prognosis with any hopes for the future. One patient, in his 60s with pancreatic cancer, told his palliative care clinician that he had already told friends he was going to die. Although his disease was stable on treatment, he kept wanting to talk about choices for hospice and how chemotherapy was unlikely to help. As he talked, his wife sat next to him looking overwhelmed.

In our experience, with either type of persistent one-sidedness the clinician should consider possible underlying and untreated anxiety or depression or other difficulty with coping, such as substance use or a trauma history. With these patients, we let the oncologist know that we are helping the patient with coping. The palliative care team should also coordinate care more frequently and ensure that the patient has enough emotional support, including social work, psychology, psychiatry, and spiritual care.

A third pattern is reflected in patients who move frequently and dramatically between very optimistic hopes and fatalistic worries. In one minute, they talk only about being cured and, in the next, about funeral arrangements. This dramatic pattern often occurs soon after diagnosis, although it can persist throughout the illness. In qualitative work, Curtis et al. found that these patients view prognostic information as a threat to hopes and prefer that clinicians, including oncologists, provide prognostic information cautiously and indirectly. In this situation, we let the oncologist know that the patient may not welcome direct prognostic information and that we are teaching the patient skills to cope with the intense thoughts and emotions of serious illness. (This coping skills approach is discussed in Chapter 3.)

Although collaboration often occurs through conversations, a written record of patients' prognostic understanding, hopes, worries, and goals is essential. We detail this information longitudinally in the health record in

Table 2.2 EXAMPLE DOCUMENTATION TEMPLATE

Illness understanding	George knows that he is not a surgical candidate, that his cancer cannot be removed.
Hopes	George is hoping for a cure through a breakthrough in immunotherapy. He hopes to be able to meet his grandchildren (his children are not yet married).
Worries	George acknowledges that a part of him worries. It is hard for him to talk specifically about his worries.
Prognostic information discussed	Discussed that it is hard to live with cancer.
What's important	He is focused on fighting the cancer and learning about experimental options.
Recommendations	Palliative care will continue to help George adapt to his illness.

a centralized advance care planning module so that all clinicians caring for the patient can document and easily view what others have discussed. Patients commonly have several conversations that develop their prognostic awareness with different clinicians, including the oncologist, primary care clinician, palliative care clinician, and hospitalist. Easy-to-find, centralized documentation of a patient's prognostic awareness allows clinicians to build on each other's work. The following template, filled in for George, is located centrally in our electronic health record (through Epic) (Table 2.2).

MEETING THE CHALLENGE OF PAIRING HOPES AND WORRIES

In this chapter, we discussed how we help patients pair hopes and worries, a critical psychological step in coping with serious illness. With patients who focus solely on hope, we align with their hopes and touch upon the illness gently. Once patients can acknowledge both hopes and worries, we reflect both back empathically. This reflection often needs only a sentence to summarize. We also reassure patients that it is normal to have a mix of thoughts and feelings related to the illness. Once patients can accept the pairing, they have met this second challenge. They will elaborate on this pairing through the next three challenges.

Occasionally, despite touching upon the illness very gently, patients struggle to acknowledge worries at all. Unlike George, these patients remain focused exclusively on optimistic hopes. With these patients, we move to the third challenge and return to pairing when they have developed more coping skills. (Patients who are hesitant to talk about the future may also need a specialist approach, detailed in Chapter 4.) The following schema shows how patients can move between these challenges.

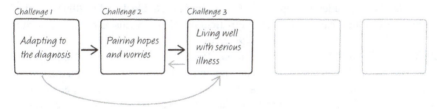

COMMUNICATION SKILLS SUMMARY

CHAPTER 1: ADAPTING TO THE DIAGNOSIS

Assess prognostic awareness: What is your understanding of your illness? Looking to the future, what are your hopes? What are your worries?

Support coping: Normalize, align, contain.

Be an interpreter: Interpret the patient for the oncologist and the oncologist for the patient.

CHAPTER 2: PAIRING HOPES AND WORRIES

For patients who focus solely on hope: Align with hope and touch upon the illness by

- empathizing
- understanding the illness's impact on others

- suggesting a worried part
- mentioning the "what ifs"
- linking to worries with "even though"

For patients who acknowledge hopes and worries: Pair the patient's hopes and worries, and normalize these mixed feelings.

FURTHER READING

Bakitas, M., Lyons, K. D., Hegel, M. T., & Ahles, T. (2013). Oncologists' perspectives on concurrent palliative care in a National Cancer Institute-designated comprehensive cancer center. *Palliative and Supportive Care, 11*(5), 415–423.

Bernacki, R., Paladino, J., Neville, B. A., Hutchings, M., Kavanagh, J., Geerse, O. P., Lakin, J., Sanders, J. J., Miller, K., Lipsitz, S., Gawande, A. A., & Block, S. D. (2019). Effect of the serious illness care program in outpatient oncology: A cluster randomized clinical trial. *JAMA Internal Medicine, 179*(6), 751–759.

Bluhm, M., Connell, C. M., De Vries, R. G., Janz, N. K., Bickel, K. E., & Silveira, M. J. (2016). Paradox of prescribing late chemotherapy: Oncologists explain. *Journal of Oncology Practice, 12*(12), e1006–e1015.Casellas-Grau, A., Ochoa, C., & Ruini, C. (2017). Psychological and clinical correlates of posttraumatic growth in cancer: A systematic and critical review. *Psycho-Oncology, 26*(12), 2007–2018.

Curtis, J. R., Engelberg, R., Young, J. P., Vig, L. K., Reinke, L. F., Wenrich, M. D., McGrath, B., McCown, E., & Back, A. L. (2008). An approach to understanding the interaction of hope and desire for explicit prognostic information among individuals with severe chronic obstructive pulmonary disease or advanced cancer. *Journal of Palliative Medicine, 11*(4), 610–620.

Dor-Ziderman, Y., Lutz, A., & Goldstein, A. (2019). Prediction-based neural mechanisms for shielding the self from existential threat. *Neuroimage, 202*, 116080.

Feros, D. L., Lane, L., Ciarrochi, J., & Blackledge, J. T. (2013). Acceptance and commitment therapy (ACT) for improving the lives of cancer patients: A preliminary study. *Psycho-Oncology, 22*(2), 459–464.

Jackson, V. A., Jacobsen, J., Greer, J. A., Pirl, W. F., Temel, J. S., & Back, A. L. (2013). The cultivation of prognostic awareness through the provision of early palliative care in the ambulatory setting: A communication guide. *Journal of Palliative Medicine, 16*(8), 894–900.

Jackson, V. A., Mack, J., Matsuyama, R., Lakoma, M. D., Sullivan, A. M., Arnold, R. M., Weeks, J. C., & Block, S. D. (2008). A qualitative study of oncologists' approaches to end-of-life care. *Journal of Palliative Medicine, 11*(6), 893–906.

Jacobsen, J., Brenner, K., Greer, J. A., Jacobo, M., Rosenberg, L., Nipp, R. D., & Jackson, V. A. (2018). When a patient is reluctant to talk about it: A dual framework to focus on living well and tolerate the possibility of dying. *Journal of Palliative Medicine, 21*(3), 322–327.

Jacobsen, J., Thomas, J. D., & Jackson, V. A. (2013). Misunderstandings about prognosis: An approach for palliative care consultants when the patient does not seem to understand what was said. *Journal of Palliative Medicine, 16*(1), 91–95.

McKay, M., Wood, J., & Brantley, J. (2007). *The dialectical behavior therapy skills workbook.* New Harbinger Publications, Inc.

Mohabbat-Bahar, S., Maleki-Rizi, F., Akbari, M. E., & Moradi-Joo, M. (2015). Effectiveness of group training based on acceptance and commitment therapy on anxiety and depression of women with breast cancer. *Iranian Journal of Cancer Prevention, 8*(2), 71–76.

Ransom, S., Sheldon, K. M., & Jacobsen, P. B. (2008). Actual change and inaccurate recall contribute to posttraumatic growth following radiotherapy. *Journal of Consulting and Clinical Psychology, 76*(5), 811–819.

Schwartz, R. C., & Sweezy, M. (2020). *Internal family systems therapy* (2nd ed.). Guildford Press.

Siegel, D. J., & Bryson, T. P. (2014). *No-drama discipline.* Bantam.

Siegel, D. J., & Bryson, T. P. (2019). *The yes brain: How to cultivate courage, curiosity, and resilience in your child.* Random House.

Thoma, N., Pilecki, B., & McKay, D. (2015). Contemporary cognitive behavior therapy: A review of theory, history, and evidence. *Psychodynamic Psychiatry, 43*(3), 423–461.

van Vliet, L., Francke, A., Tomson, S., Plum, N., van der Wall, E., & Bensing, J. (2013). When cure is no option: How explicit and hopeful can information be given? A qualitative study in breast cancer. *Patient Education and Counseling, 90*(3), 315–322.

Wright, A. A., Keating, N. L., Ayanian, J. Z., Chrischilles, E. A., Kahn, K. L., Ritchie, C. S., Weeks, J. C., Earle, C. C., & Landrum, M. B. (2016). Family perspectives on aggressive cancer care near the end of life. *Journal of the American Medical Association, 315*(3), 284–292.

Living Well with Serious Illness

Carlos, a father of two teenage children, began seeing palliative care soon after his diagnosis of metastatic colon cancer. Carlos could pair hopes and worries but was more aligned with his worries. He told us that he could not let himself feel hopeful or plan for enjoyable times. He feared looking forward to them and then being disappointed by the cancer. Now, 4 months later, his cancer has stabilized, and he says that he can trust his body. He is ready to talk about how to spend his time and "make the most of it."

THE CHALLENGE OF LIVING WELL WITH SERIOUS ILLNESS

A clinician meeting with Carlos faces a delicate task. Even though Carlos's cancer is stable on treatment, his life has been limited by the cancer and its treatment. He has taken medical leave because he no longer has the concentration and stamina for work, but he feels well most of the time. He spends his days at home while his wife is at work and his children are in school. He feels bored and lonely. Carlos faces the third challenge: living well with serious illness. Carlos, with help from his clinician, will develop goals that are both realistic and aligned with his values, and figure out how to actualize them.

Living well is about patients developing their hopes, even though their life is or will be limited by a serious illness. Early in the illness, many patients express both hopes and worries, but their hopes tend to be narrow—for a miracle cure or treatment. As clinicians, we don't need to dispute optimistic hopes; rather, we help patients expand their hopes to encompass living well now.

The expansion is indicated by the arrows pointing out from hopes into living well (Figure 3.1). The "living well" circle may still include optimistic hopes for a miracle or cure. It often includes goals to feel as well as possible physically and psychologically. It might also include connecting to loved ones or repairing relationships. Some patients take on legacy projects such as writing letters or making scrapbooks; others prefer to focus on living normally day to day. Living well also includes coping with worries so that they do not ruin the good times.

Our focus on living well also fosters clinical attunement. When we ask patients what's most important to them and help them make realistic plans for how to live well, patients see that our role includes being responsive to their need for hope and for a focus on living. One patient,

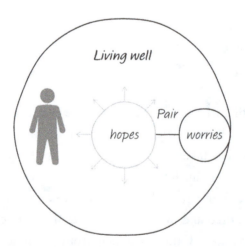

Figure 3.1 Adding challenge 3: living well with serious illness. Living well with serious illness involves helping patients to expand their hopes and learn to cope with their worries.

living with undertreated pain, was stunned when we increased his pain medication so that he could putter around on the golf course: "So your job is to help me do things and live as much as I can? That makes me so happy."

Supporting a patient's need for living well now also builds the partnership critical as the cancer advances, when we will help our patient reimagine living well. Later still, this partnership will help when the patient faces end-of-life decisions and needs our guidance through end-of-life decision-making.

In this chapter, we discuss how to help patients live well with serious illness. In contrast to optimistic, longer-term hopes, living well applies to the near future. It can and should start now. It does not rely on extraordinary medical fortune. We first discuss, from our research, how coping skills help patients live well. Then we describe the most important coping skills and how to teach them to patients. Finally, we touch on how our coping support extends to oncology colleagues.

UNDERSTANDING OUR RESEARCH ON COPING

When patients are diagnosed, they may not understand how much help they may need in learning to cope with the illness, the treatments, and the uncertainty inherent in their situation. Many prefer coping skills that have helped them manage stress in the past, such as distraction, exercise, or intellectualization. However, living well with a serious illness requires a large repertoire of coping skills.

Indeed, providing coping support is a primary mechanism by which palliative care improves patients' quality of life and mood. We had learned from multiple trials that palliative care improves quality of life and mood, but the following question remained: Which specific interventions accounted for these effects? An answer came from our large randomized controlled trial of early integrated palliative care (for patients with newly diagnosed advanced lung or non-colorectal gastrointestinal cancer). We collected detailed information on coping from patients and clinicians. Specifically, after each palliative care visit, clinicians completed a survey detailing the visit content. In the 2,921 palliative care visits with 171 study patients, clinicians most frequently addressed symptom management (74.5%) and coping (64.2%).

Patients assigned to early palliative care who had a greater proportion of visits that addressed coping reported improved quality of life and reduced depression by 24 weeks. In addition, as part of this trial, patients completed a survey several times on their use of coping skills. The survey results showed us that the early integrated palliative care intervention increased patients' use of specific coping skills that helped them face the illness. These skills included reframing the situation in a positive light, accepting the situation, and actively coping by improving the situation (for example, improving diet or calling a friend to help with grocery shopping). Moreover, the increased use of these coping skills accounted for the significant improvements in patient-reported quality of life and depression. Teaching patients coping skills is crucial for improving outcomes.

HOW TO HELP PATIENTS LIVE WELL WITH SERIOUS ILLNESS

We synthesized our research findings, a review of the literature, and our clinical experience into a three-part approach for clinicians to help patients develop coping skills: exploring the meaning of living well, strengthening patients' current coping skills, and suggesting new skills.

Explore the Meaning of Living Well with Serious Illness

Although it might be tempting to ask patients directly for their ideas on living well, setting up that conversation is essential. Even with cancer stabilized on therapy, almost all patients lose quality of life. Many patients with metastatic disease cannot work full time. Many live with physical symptoms from the cancer or the treatment. Even for asymptomatic patients, treatment consumes time and mental energy. They spend time going to clinic, getting scans, filling prescriptions, and resting and recovering after treatment. And the diagnosis itself brings the realization that time is limited. Thus, before a conversation about how to live well, we acknowledge these losses: "I can't imagine how challenging this has been." Only after empathizing can we ask, "What does it mean for you to live well with this illness?"

In the following example, a continuation of an example from Chapter 2, the clinician talks with a patient about how to live well with a prematurely shortened lifespan. Over months, the clinician gathered a sense of the patient's style and interests. She now uses this information to tailor her questions to be relevant to the patient (an example of clinical attunement).

Talking about how to live well with the illness

DIALOG	OUR PERSPECTIVE
CLINICIAN: Because it's how to live in both worlds?	
PATIENT: Yeah.	
CLINICIAN: So that is a really important thing for us to think about, because most patients who I spend time with have trouble with this whole piece of knowing that time is not going to be as long as we want. And even if I said to you, it's going to be 5 years, it's not long enough. It still feels like this is not part of what the plan was going to be.	*Acknowledges and empathizes with the patient's sadness that the life has been shortened.*
PATIENT: That's not the plan.	

Dialog	Our perspective
CLINICIAN: That's not the plan. So, the question is, what do you do with that time? And I think for a lot of people, this whole idea of "Well, just live each day to the fullest" isn't enough. How the flip am I supposed to do that? You want to be a realist because you're a business guy. You're an ops guy. You do the planning. And how do you plan for this and still live? Is that right?	*Acknowledges the patient's loss before pivoting to the question of how to live well. Explores how to live well by connecting the question to the patient's self-concept as a practical planner.*
PATIENT: Yeah, that sounds spot on.	

Because large existential questions can seem overly personal in the clinical setting, we often introduce the question of how to live well by connecting it to our clinical role: "An important part of my job is to ensure that you have the best quality of life possible. So, it is helpful for me to know what it means for you to live well with this illness. Would you talk about that?"

Patients give a wide variety of responses. Many mention wanting to feel well. Many also talk about loved ones, wanting to have good times and to ensure that loved ones are prepared. One important theme is the wish for life to be normal. As one patient said, "I cannot live every day as it if were my last. That is pretty stressful. I cannot go around looking for meaning in every moment. I just want a normal day."

Some patients have trouble responding, believing that they should focus on disease management: "How can I miss treatment to go on vacation this summer? Shouldn't I stay nearby?" Others are afraid to enjoy small pleasures. They might have adopted a strict diet or wellness program that provides hope and benefit but also impairs quality of life. A few get so overwhelmed by the diagnosis, prognosis, treatments, and loss of regular life routine that they cannot find a new joyful focus. They find only meager hopes and stay mostly fixed at worries. These patients are best supported through regular visits (at least monthly) with the palliative care clinician to focus on coping skills and should be referred to social work, psychiatry, and pastoral care as needed.

Finally, a few patients have had unexpected or late responses to treatment. They had been preparing for end of life when their disease stabilizes suddenly. Dramatic changes, even positive ones, are surprisingly hard to adapt to, and these patients can have trouble reconnecting with living for fear of being disappointed. They then feel ungrateful and guilty about not taking advantage of unexpected extra time. These lucky patients may therefore have trouble discussing living well. To ease their distress, we explain that even positive change needs adaptation and normalize this rare experience: "I often see that, when patients have unexpected recoveries like you, they feel confused. On the one hand, they can't believe their luck and feel so happy. On the other hand, they are afraid that, if they start looking forward and making plans, their future will be snatched away again. Some people feel guilty, others depressed. It can take time to readjust." As we interpret the patient's experience for the patient, we maintain attunement by mirroring how he or she swings between hopes and worries. With time and understanding, these patients trust their recovery and reengage in living.

Strengthening Existing Coping Skills

Patients have learned many ways to cope with stressors throughout their lives, ways that they bring to a serious illness. Before we teach new skills, we aim to strengthen patients' existing coping skills by initially reminding them of their skills: "How have you coped with difficult situations in the past?" Then we explore how they are currently coping: "How have you coped with this illness? What have you been doing to get through these tough times?" Patients can be unaware of their coping strategies. In this case, focused questions help elicit their strategies. Our early integrated palliative care encounters included several examples:

- "Are you going to watch any of the Olympics? Does that interest you?"
- "Besides fixing things, what else do you like to do?"
- "Before, when you were feeling well and not dealing with this kind of crap on your plate, what would you like to do? How did you spend your time?"

We learn whether patients rely on just one or two strategies or use a range and whether they rely on coping strategies that soon will be limited by the illness, such as working or exercise. We also learn how aware patients are of their coping. Some can readily explain their different strategies to manage their stress. Others need us to give examples of strategies. We might say, "Some people cope by trying to think positively and keep up their hopes. Is this something that is helpful for you?" These patients, who are less aware of their coping, need new strategies introduced slowly.

As patients explain how they are coping, we name and contextualize the strategies: "It sounds like one way that you cope is by distracting yourself and thinking about other things. Distraction is a powerful way manage the stress of an illness. The break gives you needed energy." In the assessment, we also listen for disengaged, potentially harmful strategies such as substance use or social withdrawal. We then involve social work and the rest of the interdisciplinary team.

To provide a vocabulary to help with the coping assessment, we now detail diverse, effective coping skills. Their diversity helps patients manage thoughts and feelings at different times, with different people, and under different circumstances. The skills are divided into four groups: (1) behavioral, (2) cognitive, (3) emotional, and (4) existential (Table 3.1), although some skills fit into more than one group.

Table 3.1 COPING SKILLS

Skill	Example
BEHAVIORAL	
Focusing on the body	• Using relaxation strategies • Maintaining good sleep • Exercising
Collaborative problem solving	• Planning a feasible trip given a need for supplemental oxygen
Seeking social support	• Determining which friends and family can provide what support
COGNITIVE	
Distraction	• Doing puzzles, watching TV
Intellectualization	• Thinking about facts and details
Positive reframing	• Considering positive life changes from the illness • Comparing oneself with those less fortunate
Cognitive restructuring	• Identifying and refuting irrational or maladaptive thoughts
Self-efficacy	• Believing in oneself and refraining from self-blame
EMOTIONAL	
Enhancing positive emotions	• Focusing on moments of joy and happiness • Helping others laugh • Expressing appreciation and gratitude
Maintaining/redirecting hope	• Expanding hopes to include more attainable hopes
Mindfulness	• Observing emotions and thoughts without trying change them
EXISTENTIAL	
Making meaning	• Reflecting on one's experiences and legacy • Joining or starting a community effort
Incorporating religion or spirituality	• Praying • Attending church services • Connecting with nature
Finding acceptance	• Finding emotional, cognitive, and behavioral equanimity

BEHAVIORAL SKILLS

In the category of behavioral skills, patients alleviate stress by taking action. The skills are focusing on the body, collaborative problem solving, and seeking social support. These skills are summarized in Table 3.2 at the end of this section.

Focusing on the Body

This overall skill includes relaxation strategies, such as deep breathing and progressive muscle relaxation. It also includes good sleep, exercise, nutrition, and hygiene. Such strategies are often familiar to patients and their assessment can happen in the palliative care symptom assessment.

As the illness progresses, patients' capacity to build new habits, even in these familiar domains, may get strained. Patients frustrated by fatigue or pain should be encouraged to take breaks when learning new habits. Making micro changes helps—for example, adding 10 minutes of exercise or 1 minute of meditation. These less ambitious, more achievable behavioral changes are more likely to stick. Once integrated into the patient's routine, they can expand in length or intensity.

Collaborative Problem Solving

With a serious illness, patients face a multitude of new problems, ranging from the practical (getting to appointments) to the existential (living with uncertainty). When our patient identifies a problem, we brainstorm and plan a solution together so that the potential solution reflects both the patient's values and the medical realities. For instance, for an oxygen-dependent patient who has long wanted to travel, we might brainstorm local rather than overseas destinations. Solving problems together is an important way that we build the partnership on which we will draw later in the illness when patients face end-of-life decisions.

Collaborative problem-solving was important with Carlos. His cancer was stable on treatment for a long time. Although he couldn't work because of fatigue, he otherwise felt well. However, this good outcome also left Carlos with much time alone and no activities or goals outside of attending medical appointments. In our visits, he talked about his frustration and how he wanted a place to go and something to do.

As we talked about possible solutions, Carlos had an idea: He decided to buy a motorcycle, something he would never have bought before his illness. As a father, he wanted to stay safe, but the risks now mattered less, and motorcycle riding was an enjoyable activity that he could do despite his fatigue. The motorcycle also created new social interactions, as Carlos spent hours hanging out at the repair shop. He described his motorcycle as the one small benefit of his cancer.

The lesson is to brainstorm together ways to adjust activities to patients' level of function, especially as their physical status declines. At the same time, as clinicians, we should remain attuned to patients' need to grieve the loss of prior function before we suggest new activities. Otherwise, the brainstorming and problem solving can invalidate patients' illness experience.

In the next example, the patient has identified a problem, that her husband won't talk about the possibility of her dying. The clinician collaborates in problem solving by asking questions and reflecting back what has been said.

Encouraging collaborative problem solving

CLINICIAN: Is there any other way to help prepare him or make sure that he's as supported as he can be when you're gone?

PATIENT: I don't know what else to do. I've sat him down. I've talked with him. I've said, "And I'm not going to be here forever." And my girlfriend keeps telling me, "He's going to hear your words."

CLINICIAN: Yeah, because you've sat him down and you've said that to him.

PATIENT: Yeah. Over and over.

CLINICIAN: Good. Have you written anything to him?

PATIENT: No.

CLINICIAN: Do you like to write? Are you a—not so much?

PATIENT: No, not so much. Yeah, I suppose I could. I mean, I don't see why not. I could. I never thought of it, truthfully.

CLINICIAN: Just something to think about. Because what I imagine you might want is for him to hold your love and the support that you've been giving him, when things are tough for him later.

Seeking Social Support

Encouraging patients to seek social support is a variation of collaborative problem solving. We help patients reflect on the different categories of social support that they need, such as informational, practical, or emotional, and on who could meet those needs. For example, for information support: Who could offer advice and information? For practical support: Who could help with day-to-day tasks such as making meals, getting to appointments, or going shopping? For emotional support: Who could empathize and listen to the experience of life-limiting cancer? Patients have rarely differentiated the types of social support and often appreciate learning about these categories. The categorization also helps clinicians, patients, and families to identify and fill gaps in support.

In the following example, the clinician helps a patient think through her different types of social support, specifically how to engage her husband, her daughter Jenny, and her friend Susan.

Differentiating sources of social support

CLINICIAN: I think that you've got a husband who is totally committed to you and loyal and will try to give anything you need. But this piece about being a sounding board for the illness—probably not so much. And for your daughter Jenny too; it's not a role you want to put her in right now. The other thing I hear is that you've got a lot of internal resources to do some of this yourself, the journaling. But I think having your friend Susan, as another person that you can do this with, is huge.

PATIENT: I have very good support.

The preceding example illustrates how we educate patients about sources of social support. Patients can then more effectively ask for help. In the next example, the clinician discusses a seemingly paradoxical kind of social support, that some patients prefer to see only their closest friends.

Preferring less social support

CLINICIAN: What I'm hearing you say is you've got this huge circle of people, used to being very active, and now your instincts are just to hunker down and be more by yourself.

PATIENT: You know, people have come out of the dark, have insisted on seeing me, and I was just like, "Guys, you know, you're once a year."

CLINICIAN: One thing that I say is, with a serious illness, there's what I call orbits. There's the inner orbit of people. With them, you might not have brushed your teeth and you're still in your pajamas, and it's fine that they come over. They are the people who should be around now. It's really about them. You shouldn't feel guilty and think that you need to hang out with someone whom you haven't seen in a year, right?

PATIENT: Yup.

CLINICIAN: It's all about surrounding yourself with people who help you feel better.

Table 3.2 OPERATIONALIZING BEHAVIORAL SKILLS WITH PATIENTS

Behavioral Skill	Steps in Operationalizing the Skill*
Body-focused strategies	1. Ask about habits or previous experience (sleep, exercise, nutrition, hygiene, mindfulness, or meditation). 2. Work with the patient to set a goal. 3. Consider whether a micro change could help achieve the goal.
Collaborative problem solving	1. Jointly identify a problem related to the illness. 2. Consider the medical context and what is possible. 3. Explore the patient's values related to the problem. 4. Brainstorm possible solutions. 5. Jointly develop a plan.
Seeking social support	1. Ask about the patient's social support with attention to the three types (informational, practical, emotional). 2. Jointly consider any gaps and brainstorm strategies for filling them.

*Remember to document the plan or goal and follow up at the next visit.

COGNITIVE SKILLS

In the category of cognitive skills, patients ease stress by changing their thoughts. The skills are distraction, intellectualization, positive reframing, cognitive restructuring, and self-efficacy. Unlike behavior-focused skills, which are familiar and easy for patients to incorporate, some of the cognitive skills require teaching and practice. With unfamiliar skills, we first model the skill, then name what we did, and finally encourage the patient to use the skill at home (Table 3.3).

Distraction

This skill entails diverting attention toward thoughts or behaviors unrelated to the illness. Common methods of distraction include watching TV, playing games, reading, exercising, or working. Many patients use this skill instinctively. When patients are using this skill, we name it and explain that it's healthy: "It sounds like you can take a break from all of this by playing with your grandchildren. Distracting yourself is a healthy way to cope." When a patient needs but has forgotten about distraction, we encourage and name it: "It can be helpful for patients to have times when they forget about the cancer. What are ways that you distract yourself from this?" (Distraction does not fit neatly into the four-part categorization. It is both cognitive and behavioral—patients can *think about* or *do* something else.)

In the following example, the clinician gives the patient permission to stop talking about the illness and to focus on daily activities.

Giving permission to use distraction

CLINICIAN: The thing is, you don't have to talk about this illness all the time. You can say to people, "Guys, today I just want to watch the game," because your life cannot be only this illness. You are more than this illness.

PATIENT: Yeah, I agree with you.

CLINICIAN: You can show them how to do that. They'll follow your lead. If you say, "Oh, I'm feeling anxious about it, and I just feel like shit," then they'll need to meet you there. But it's okay to have days when you say, "You know what? I don't really want to talk about that. Can we just go for a walk, or let's go watch the game," or whatever else takes your mind away. Distraction doesn't mean that you're not being a responsible adult with the illness. It's okay to have times when you say, "I'm just going to put that away, and we'll deal with it another time."

In the next example, the clinician explores and names how a patient is coping by using distraction.

Exploring healthy distraction

PATIENT: If I'm in really tough shape, I spend a lot of time watching bird cams. And those birds cams show the—in this case, it was owls and eagles—show the nesting pair. They lay the eggs. Then the eggs hatch. And then the chicks grow up. And then they fledge. And it's a very long process, a couple months, but it's completely interesting. And it is something I can do when I feel just awful.

CLINICIAN: What do you think draws you to that? It's great.

PATIENT: It's out of my comfort zone. It's something I don't know anything about, and it's life. It's life from beginning to getting out of the nest. And it has symbolism to my kids. It has symbolism about my situation. So it's just a lovely thing to do, and it's mindless. To be honest, it's pretty mindless.

CLINICIAN: So what I hear you say is that you have different strategies that you use, depending upon what's happening in your world, and that you've been able to adapt because sometimes the cancer makes you feel crummy. And other days, you feel really pretty much like yourself or more like yourself. And I hear that distraction is one strategy.

PATIENT: Distraction's huge when I don't feel well.

CLINICIAN: Say more about that.

PATIENT: I play a lot of smartphone games. They all think I'm obsessed [laughter], but what it does is actually just take my mind off of things. And then if I'm really fatigued, what I'll do is, if I don't feel like really sleeping, instead of lying there thinking about gloom and doom, I will listen to podcasts. And that helps a lot.

CLINICIAN: And so, just even with the birds and with the podcasts, it's a way to sort of be engaged and learn and grow in something that you may not know something about, but it doesn't require you to feel sharp and on point enough to digest a book, like a memoir or something like that.

PATIENT: Right. I can listen to somebody else talk and just get into their moment as opposed to being in mine.

Intellectualization

This skill entails avoiding uncomfortable emotion by focusing on facts or logic related to the illness—in general, using thinking about the illness to avoid feeling. In contrast to distraction, in which patients take their mind away from the illness, with intellectualization, patients focus on nonemotional thoughts about the illness, typically through planning, organizing, or researching.

When patients are overwhelmed, we mention this skill: "It sounds like there are times during the day when you can feel very sad. Sometimes patients find it helpful to think about the details of the situation to lessen their emotions. You could organize your medications, make appointments, or even tackle your financial plans. It's healthy to have ways to stay engaged with the problem of this illness that don't make you too upset."

This skill is also useful for palliative care clinicians, who often apply it at the end of difficult family meetings: "We are going to come back tomorrow morning. Before then, it sounds like your plan is to call your family and make an inventory of what you might need when you go home." The concrete details of plans and next steps shift the focus for all of us away from the emotions of a difficult conversation.

Although helpful, this skill is often overused. For example, in difficult family meetings, patients, family members, and even clinicians can easily pay too much attention to medical and logistical details and too little attention to their own emotions. This focus on details prevents a focus on emotion or meaning and can mean avoiding the implications of the illness and prognosis. When we observe patients overusing this skill, we help them shift their focus from facts to feelings.

For example, Henry, in his mid-40s with young children and metastatic lung cancer, used mostly intellectualization. He talked about treatment options with his clinicians, read on the internet, and made financial plans for his family. He showed little emotion related to the illness. Using this approach, Henry adapted to the diagnosis and continued his work and family routines. However, when we asked about his goals for living well, Henry mentioned his wife was very angry about his illness and wondered how to help her.

In our conversation, we discussed how it can be important for patients and families to share their grief and other feelings. We encouraged Henry to talk about his feelings with his wife, even though these conversations would feel uncomfortable. Over time, in conversations with his wife, Henry identified and talked about his deep sadness. He was sad for himself and for his children, who would not have his guidance. Recognizing these feelings alleviated Henry's unacknowledged loneliness and helped him connect with his wife, who was grateful to grieve with Henry. Our role with patients is not insight-oriented psychotherapy, but we can encourage patients to experience rather than ignore the normal (difficult) feelings related to their illness.

Positive Reframing
This skill entails seeing matters in a more positive light or looking for good aspects. Some patients find good aspects by comparing themselves to hypothetical others with perceived worse circumstances. One patient with an unresectable glioblastoma told us that if he had pancreatic cancer, he would suffer more pain. Another patient with a rapid disease trajectory observed that, if he had been hit by a bus, he would not have had time to say goodbye to his family.

Other patients find positive consequences that are independent of the circumstances of others, such as increased family cohesion or the caring outreach and support offered by friends. One patient told us how she never knew how loved she was until she got sick. Another described how he had never taken the time to enjoy nature until the illness forced him to slow down.

Clinicians can notice and name these reframings: "I hear you imagining an even worse situation. Reframing your situation in a positive light is a healthy way to cope." Or, "It sounds like even though this illness has been so difficult, you have been able to find good things. Finding positives is a healthy way to cope with a difficult situation."

We also invite patients to use this skill, first acknowledging how difficult the illness experience has been (patients need us to be able to see their emotional pain before exploring the situation's positive aspects): "These past few months have been so hard. I wonder also—has there been any-thing good coming from this diagnosis?"

Cognitive Restructuring

Cancer diagnosis and treatment brings forth cognitive distortions. Examples include all-or-nothing thinking (for example, thinking that one can be happy only once the cancer is cured) and catastrophizing (thinking that one will die much sooner than the expected prognosis or die in pain or become addicted to opioids). Modeling the skill of cognitive restruc-turing, the clinician identifies and disputes irrational or maladaptive thoughts in order to help patients reframe an admittedly difficult situation more realistically.

For example, a common maladaptive thought is that the cancer will grow faster on dose-reduced chemotherapy (all-or-nothing thinking). To dispute this (and many a) maladaptive thought, a useful phrase is, "I wonder." "I wonder whether, in the back of your mind, you are thinking that only the full dose of chemotherapy will work?" If the patient agrees, we ask more: "Can you tell me more about what you are thinking about the dose?" Next, we empathize with the patient: "This uncertainty is so hard." Finally, we invite the patient to consider a contrary view by linking it to the patient's perspective using the "and" conjunction (not "but"). For example, "I hear you are very worried that reducing the chemotherapy is going to make the cancer grow. And what we know is that each person metabolizes chemotherapy differently. A lower dose may be as effective as a higher dose, just with fewer side effects."

Another common maladaptive thought is that thinking about the prognosis, or "being negative," will make the cancer worse or ruin good times (another example of all-or-nothing thinking). Patients are often told by well-meaning friends and family, "You have to be positive or the cancer will grow." To dispute this misconception by introducing a contrary view, we might say: "I hear you want to stay positive. And re-search tells us that negative thoughts are okay. Positive thinking does not help people live longer and patients feel less anxious when they can talk about worries."

With any maladaptive thought, even once patients identify it as mal-adaptive, they may need to dispute it more than once. We anticipate this process: "It sounds like you often worry that the cancer will grow faster if you don't stay positive. It is common for unhelpful thoughts to come back. Keep reminding yourself that it is helpful to acknowledge worries."

Self-efficacy

Some patients already think, "I can get through this," or "This is re-ally hard. I am doing the best that I can." Other patients need help to develop an internal self-efficacy dialog; we then ask how they approached past difficulties. In these discussions, patients often reveal a unique tenacity or inner strength, which we highlight: "It sounds like you have a small voice inside telling you that you can make it through hard times. It also sounds like that voice is kind to you when you are struggling. Believing in yourself and not blaming yourself are healthy ways to cope."

A few patients need more explicit encouragement: "You shared with me how you organized and rallied your family to support your mom when she was sick. I was impressed by how you did that. I wonder if you could do that now for yourself, so that everyone can know what is happening with your cancer?" We also cite examples of the patient's suc-cessful coping that we have witnessed: "Although you have not faced this situation before, I have seen you be so effective in making a good quality of life. Remember after your radiation? You felt terrible, but you did all these things to feel better. You took the summer off, you swam in the pool, you had the kids cooking for you each night. Making small changes to feel better could help here too. What do you think?" Finally, we remind patients to avoid self-blame. Rather than saying, "Don't blame yourself," we tell them what to do: "Everyone struggles with this. Some of my patients find it helpful to repeat to themselves, 'This feels hard be-cause it *is* hard. I am doing the best I can.'"

Table 3.3 Operationalizing Cognitive Skills with Patients

Cognitive Skill	Steps in Operationalizing the Skill
Distraction	1. Observe how the patient is using this skill, and name it. 2. Ask, "How do you distract yourself from this illness?" 3. Explain that taking a break from thinking about the illness is healthy.
Intellectualization	*For patients overusing intellectualization:* 1. Name or explore feelings and empathize with the patient's experience. 2. Encourage the patient to talk about feelings with loved ones. *For patients who could use intellectualization to manage strong feelings:* 1. Acknowledge the strong feelings. 2. Explain that focusing on thoughts can help manage strong feelings. 3. Brainstorm how the patient might focus on nonemotional thoughts about the illness, typically through planning, organizing, or researching.
Positive reframing	*For patients already using this skill:* • Name and encourage it. *For patients not using this skill:* 1. Acknowledge the difficulty of the illness experience. 2. Invite the patient to reflect on positive aspects of the illness.
Cognitive restructuring	1. Identify a cognitive distortion. 2. Bring up the cognitive distortion gently ("I wonder if you feel that you need to stay positive to beat this cancer?"). 3. Explore the patient's perspective. 4. Empathize. 5. Invite the patient to consider a contrary view by linking it to the patient's perspective with "and."
Self-efficacy	1. Ask about past challenges and how the patient approached them. 2. Help the patient to avoid self-blame by encouraging empathy for oneself.

EMOTIONAL SKILLS

Our category of emotional skills includes enhancing positive emotions, maintaining/redirecting hope, and mindfulness (Table 3.4).

Enhancing Positive Emotions

Patients can alleviate anxiety, anger, and fear by cultivating positive emotions such as gratitude, joy, and even anticipation. Positive emotions not only counteract negative emotions, they also make patients (and all of us) more flexible, creative, integrative, and open to new information and experiences. And they build enduring resources such as social connection, knowledge, insight, and physical reserve. Take a patient who watches a funny TV show, feels energized, and goes for a walk. He bumps into a neighbor, and they start chatting. The neighbor later brings over a book that the patient might enjoy. The physical reserve (from the walk), the social resources (connection with his neighbor), and the intellectual resources (the book) can be drawn upon later.

Clinicians can help patients cultivate positive emotions by inviting discussions that elicit joy, gratitude, and happiness: "What's been good?" "What are you looking forward to?" Or, more elaborately, we might say, "Although none of us would ever want you to have cancer, I have found that some people learn valuable things about themselves and others as they cope with the disease. Has this happened for you?" Alternatively, if patients mention something or someone for which they are grateful, we ask follow-up questions, sustaining or even amplifying those feelings.

Positive emotions can also be enhanced through humor. In our transcripts, we saw many examples, which may seem counterintuitive or inappropriate with a serious illness. However, with the right timing and awareness of the patient's coping style, humor can be bonding. Here are a few examples:

- "Yeah, you're stuck with us. That's what I would say. You can fire us. But short of that, we keep coming back, like a bad penny."
- "Well, part of my job is to make sure that you don't become a junkie. (laughter) That's why they pay me."

- "She's fresh. For the love of God, doesn't she know you have cancer? Is there no love or respect?"

Fostering positive emotion was particularly important for Carlos (introduced at the start of the chapter). Toward the middle of his illness, he developed a small bowel obstruction, making it impossible to eat. His peritoneal disease precluded surgery, and he was treated with a venting G-tube and total parenteral nutrition. Fortunately, Carlos had a strong performance status. He and his clinical team hoped that a new chemotherapy would undo his blockage. After a few months, his new chemotherapy did halt the progression of his cancer, but the blockage remained. Carlos experienced his inability to eat as a severe deprivation. He loved food. He loved the social atmosphere of meals, and he suffered tremendously without them.

In our clinic visits, we empathized. Each meal was a hardship for Carlos and for his family, who did not know how to comfort him and who felt guilty eating their own meals. We suggested that we together identify and magnify the aspects of Carlos's life that did give him joy. By focusing on them, he might live more easily without normal eating.

Carlos remembered that, when his teenage children were younger, he loved board games. We encouraged him to play these now and to find other positive activities. He also loved sparkling water, which he could still drink. We encouraged him to enjoy it, perhaps experimenting with flavors and brands. We suggested that he brainstorm and list anything that helped him enjoy a small part of life. Each day he could pick an activity from the list. We also asked him to keep a daily log of his activities, so that we could talk about them at our next visit.

For scheduling reasons, we next saw Carlos after three months. His log was thick with daily activities. He had found the exercise helpful, and his family was grateful to have small ways of making him happy. And he was ready to ditch the log: "I think I got this. I think I can stop writing it down." (This example also illustrates collaborative problem solving and the promotion of self-efficacy. In practice, many coping skills overlap.)

Maintaining/Redirecting Hope

Hope, consistently identified by patients and families as critical for coping with serious illness, is nurtured when clinicians take a deep interest in what patients are hoping for. This interest can be manifested by exploring a particular hope ("Tell me more about what you are hoping for") or by asking about a range of hopes ("I hear that you are hoping for a miracle. That would be wonderful. What else are you hoping for?"). We should spend time here. We sometimes think of it as the land of hope, as a reminder to ourselves to explore. Once we understand a patient's hopes, we can align by repeating them back: "It would be wonderful to have that kind of miracle."

Even when we understand the importance of hope, we might worry, particularly as patients become sicker, that aligning with optimistic hopes would give false hope and prevent patients from making realistic plans. However, even as patients become sicker the pendulum model remains useful: As long as patients can swing to worries, supporting even optimistic hopes is beneficial, providing patients with comfort and coping support. (For patients who cannot acknowledge worries, we try to pair them, as described in Chapter 2, or go to the specialist approach of Chapter 4.) The following clinical example illustrates how to support optimistic hopes.

The patient, a young man with an aggressive sarcoma, told a newly trained palliative care clinician that hope was very important to him and that she should always be hopeful. She wanted to do so, she replied, but wondered what to do if his illness worsened and she did not have good news. The patient asked for honesty tempered with empathy: "I want you to be honest and tell me what is happening. I just want to know that you are still hoping for a cure." The clinician, grateful for a way to be honest and stay connected with the patient, was able to say: "There is nothing I would love more than a cure for your cancer."

Mindfulness

This skill entails bringing attention to thoughts and feelings in the present moment, while not judging them. Touching on cognitive, behavioral, and emotional coping, mindfulness practice helps patients develop awareness, tolerance, and even acceptance of strong feelings. Although many associate this skill with meditation or yoga, it need not be so formal: Patients can begin by using sight, sound, smell, and touch to orient to the present moment.

We explore whether patients are already using present-moment awareness: "Do you have any quick ways to relieve stress when you are on the go? Some people take a deep breath. Some look at something beautiful, something in nature, or even a bright color. Others might take a sip of water or eat a piece of chocolate very slowly." We also explore whether they have practiced mindfulness skills more specifically and mention these skills' value in serious illness. For patients new to mindfulness, we recommend a 10-minute body scan or mindful yoga practice, such as ones offered by Jon Kabat-Zinn (https://www.youtube.com/watch?v=8HYLyuJZKno).

Table 3.4 OPERATIONALIZING EMOTIONAL SKILLS WITH PATIENTS

Emotional Skill	Steps in Operationalizing the Skill
Enhancing positive emotions	1. Invite discussions that elicit gratitude or happiness.
	2. Encourage patient to make a menu of activities that help them feel better and to log these activities daily.
	3. Use humor.
Maintaining/ redirecting hope	1. Have curiosity about the patient's hopes.
	2. Ask the patient to tell you more.
	3. Ask about other hopes.
	4. Repeat back the hopes.
Mindfulness	1. Discuss informal quick ways to relieve stress, such as taking a deep breath or looking at nature.
	2. Ask the patient about mindfulness or meditation and encourage (re)starting.
	3. Recommend brief online videos.

EXISTENTIAL SKILLS

In the existential skills category, patients reflect upon their lives by making meaning, incorporating religion or spirituality, or finding acceptance (Table 3.5).

Making Meaning

This concept's modern origins began with the work of Viktor Frankl, psychiatrist and death camp survivor. His book *Man's Search for Meaning* explored the idea that our deepest motivation is discovering meaning in life. Frankl proposed that meaning can be found under all circumstances, even the most tragic. Indeed, patients with advanced cancer who reflect on meaningful moments improve their quality of life and sense of well-being, while reducing anxiety and the desire for a hastened death.

To encourage patients to use this coping skill, we ask them to reflect on their life story ("What have you liked best about your life so far?"), experiences ("What have been the most influential experiences in your life?"), legacy ("What you feel most proud of?"), and on how to spend their remaining time ("What are your big priorities for this phase of your life?").

This life review might prompt patients to write letters to loved ones, complete unfinished tasks, and reconcile relationships with family and friends. Some patients complete a creative or artistic project, such as a scrapbook, a personal history, or a quilt or woodworking project that represents their love for others. One formal approach to reflecting on one's legacy is dignity therapy, a structured reflective interview that is transcribed for patients into a legacy document.

Patients also find meaning through making a contribution. A contribution might be small, such as paying somebody a compliment or picking up an extra bottle of water. We occasionally explore this form of making meaning: "I have noticed a lot of kindness between cancer patients. I think it is because they feel for each other. I wonder if this is something you have experienced?" Some patients seek to make larger contributions, such as raising money for cancer treatment or speaking about their illness experience to trainees or support groups. We then highlight the contribution and skill: "It is wonderful that you are getting a team together to raise money for cancer. Doing something to help others is a very powerful way to cope."

Incorporating Religion or Spirituality

The majority of patients consider themselves spiritual or religious, often relying on their beliefs, practices, and communities of faith to cope with cancer. Positive spiritual and religious coping includes seeking a stronger connection with a deity or higher power and is associated with higher quality of life and better mental health. However, religiousness is also associated with lower rates of completing a living will and a greater likelihood of receiving intensive life-prolonging medical care near death. The underlying mechanisms for these associations remain unclear.

Many patients also struggle in this area. In one study, 44% of patients reported spiritual struggle or pain. This negative religious coping is evident when patients say that they are feeling punished or abandoned by God and is correlated with psychological distress, suicidal ideation, and worse quality of life.

Although most patients with advanced cancer believe that their medical team ought to address spiritual concerns, such care is often lacking, making screening for spiritual needs and referrals to pastoral care important components of early integrated palliative care.

There are several valuable tools for taking a spiritual or religious history. One is Puchalski's FICA, which stands for the following four questions:

1. Faith and belief: "What is your faith or belief?"
2. Importance: "Is it important in your life?"
3. Community: "Are you a part of a religious or spiritual community?"
4. Address in care: "How would you like to me address these issues in your health care?"

In the following example, a palliative care clinician talks with a patient who has "new age" spiritual beliefs. The patient shares her beliefs about the afterlife and the clinician validates those beliefs, encouraging the patient to cope using them.

Exploring spiritual beliefs

CLINICIAN: We haven't talked about this yet. When you think about at some point dying from this illness, is karma part of that?

PATIENT: Oh, yeah.

CLINICIAN: And is there rebirth or reincarnation in some way? Do you have a thought about that?

PATIENT: I think it's just a being. Just kind of—well, I certainly think that there's something outside the physical. It was a very difficult transition to make. But I feel the presence of people that aren't in my life anymore.

CLINICIAN: That you're still in a relationship with them in some tangible way.

Finding Acceptance

Over time patients can develop acceptance. They then seem to swing less dramatically on the pendulum. Their hopes are more realistic, and their understanding is deeper and steadier.

Acceptance has cognitive, emotional, and behavioral components. A patient who understands the prognosis (cognitive acceptance) may act as if the illness weren't happening (behavioral nonacceptance), not telling loved ones about the diagnosis. Similarly, one patient spoke at length with his palliative care clinician about his funeral (cognitive acceptance). But when he saw his oncologist later that day, he pounded the desk, angry that he would never be a father (emotional nonacceptance).

We can help by exploring the three components. When we offer patients a safe venue to ask about the disease and clarify uncertainties, we guide them toward cognitive acceptance. When we respond empathically and invite patients to talk about feelings, they develop emotional acceptance. When we help patients determine what is within their control and how they might adapt to limitations, they develop behavioral acceptance.

Acceptance takes time, lots of time, and patients need not approve or "be okay" with the illness. They can accept the likely outcome and still think that it stinks—which is why "CANCER SUCKS" T-shirts are so popular.

In the following example, a clinician celebrates a patient for enjoying life, which leads the patient to reflect on his deepening acceptance.

Recognizing acceptance

CLINICIAN: You've had a blast this summer!

PATIENT: I know it.

CLINICIAN: And it's great.

PATIENT: I can't let it get to me.

CLINICIAN: But not everybody does that, my friend.

PATIENT: Well, I accepted it, that's why. And I realize I can't beat it, but I can mess around with it.

CLINICIAN: And you can have a hell of a lot of fun until it's your time. That's exactly right.

PATIENT: Yeah.

CLINICIAN: The thing I always say is, "People who are good copers don't know that they are good copers." Because a lot of people spend a lot of time and energy saying, "This can't be true. It can't be true. I can't think it." I think that takes energy away from being able to do the fun stuff. But you said, "This is what it is, man. We're going to do our thing, and hope we get a big, long run."

PATIENT: Yeah, we'll see how long. I don't know what the long run is. But if somebody told me it'd be for three or four years, I'd take it.

Table 3.5 OPERATIONALIZING EXISTENTIAL SKILLS WITH PATIENTS

Existential Skill	Steps in Operationalizing the Skill
Making meaning	1. Encourage the patient to reflect on experiences and legacy.
	2. Invite the patient to do life review work such as writing letters, completing unfinished tasks, and reconciling relationships.
	3. Listen for and highlight the patient's community contributions.
Incorporating religion or spirituality	1. Ask about a patient's faith.
	2. Explore its importance.
	3. Ask about any involvement in a spiritual community.
	4. Ask how the patient's faith should be incorporated into health care.
Finding acceptance	1. Encourage cognitive acceptance by talking about the illness and prognosis.
	2. Encourage emotional acceptance through empathy.
	3. Encourage behavioral acceptance by considering how to adapt to or overcome limitations.

Introducing a New Skill

Having considered the whole range of coping skills and which ones the patient is already using, we next consider where the patient is in the disease trajectory and select skills to introduce. Early in the illness, research and our clinical experience support teaching behavioral skills such as problem solving and focusing on the body (getting enough sleep, eating well, and, if possible, engaging in some form of exercise). This focus on action gives patients more control of a new situation. Once patients have adapted to the diagnosis (the first challenge), we increasingly teach cognitive and emotional skills. These skills help patients maintain some control over their thoughts and feelings as the illness progresses and they have less control over their bodies, whether due to pain, fatigue, or their ongoing treatment. Once patients have had time to live with and consider the meaning of the prognosis (the fourth challenge), we increasingly consider existential skills.

When introducing new skills we also consider the diversity of the patient's skills because the four coping skills categories—behavioral, cognitive, emotional, and existential—work synergistically. For example, many patients experience less stress if they exercise while listening to music. Exercise relaxes the body and music deepens the relaxation response by shifting the focus to the present moment. When a patient uses skills from just one category, we therefore suggest a skill from a different category.

As we found in our research and clinical practice, certain coping skills are particularly important to help patients manage the emotions around accurate prognostic awareness. Specifically, among patients with accurate prognostic awareness, those who take action to make things better (a variety of problem solving) or look for something good (positive reframing) experience a higher quality of life and mood than patients who do not use these skills.

Interestingly, patients with inaccurately optimistic perceptions (low prognostic awareness) also experience a high quality of life and mood. Denial may be an effective coping strategy, at least in the short term, but it leaves patients unprepared to make medical decisions when they get sicker. Thus, when patients are struggling to cope with the prognosis, we consider introducing the skills of problem solving and positive reframing.

For all patients, we often introduce new coping skills when they feel stuck or unhappy about a specific event or situation. Jessica had come to clinic overwhelmed and frustrated because her longtime oncologist was retiring. We empathized and asked about her feelings. As she described her frustrations, we listened for any positive aspects. Jessica spontaneously acknowledged her oncologist for his experience and outstanding clinical care. Once Jessica was less frustrated, we suggested a positive reframe: "It is frustrating to lose a trusted clinician and it sounds like you were lucky to have your oncologist. I wonder: Is it possible that there are any positives in this situation?" Jessica then mentioned the advantages of her new clinician, who was less clinically busy and a better emotional match for her. We then summarized the skill: "Sometimes the best that you can do is just to look for the good things in all this stuff that we wish weren't happening."

We also introduce new skills when a patient's long-time coping skill may soon become limited by the illness. Janet, a 52-year-old teacher with metastatic lung cancer, was an avid runner. She had struggled with her weight in her early 20s, and running had given her control over her appearance and freed her to enjoy eating. The more that she ran, the more benefits she noticed. She coped better with stress and, through the local running group, had developed her social network.

Now she could run only at the end of each chemotherapy cycle. When she talked of returning to her running routine, we worried that she would need other skills to cope with stress and find connection as she became sicker.

When patients have relied on a single skill now limited by the illness, we ask them to identify what was most important about it. Exercise, for example, offers many benefits, including physical and mental relaxation, distraction, and social connection. Janet eventually identified what she missed most: the stress relief. She loved how she felt after a long run. Through our conversation, Janet realized that she could relieve stress also through gentle stretching. Although not her first choice, she adopted this new skill.

If Janet had identified distraction as the key component, we would have brainstormed lower-intensity alternatives such as movies, knitting, or puzzles. If the meditative aspect of exercise had been important, we could have considered a breathing meditation.

Expanding a patient's coping repertoire has short- and long-term advantages. In the short term, the new skills help patients release negative emotions, feel relief, and manage daily living. In the long term, they improve patients' capacity for the challenges of disease progression, such as legacy work, saying goodbye, and making amends. In addition, learning new coping skills, even amidst loss, helps patients see that even illness can be a source of growth and hope.

An occasional homework assignment can solidify a new coping skill. We tend to assign a homework log (as we did for Carlos) with skills that enhance positive emotion or focus on the body. We remember (with a note in the chart) to check on the log at the next visit! Following up signals our belief in the intervention and fosters its use.

Patients to whom we assign this task are usually struggling to cultivate positive emotions, often due to depression, and need a lot of support to try a new coping skill. One young patient could make a change only after his depression had been treated and only with one new micro skill at a time. For example, his assignment one week was just to sit in the sun for 10 minutes daily. Only once he could do this regularly did we together pick a new goal, taking a short walk with his wife.

Tips for Helping Patients Live Well with Serious Illness

WHY

A focus on living well helps patients feel better and cope with their illness.

WHEN

Begin after patients have adjusted to the diagnosis and are in a treatment routine with symptoms controlled. Patients need not have met the second challenge of pairing hopes and worries in order to focus on living well.

HOW

Promote healthy coping by
- exploring what it means to live well with serious illness.
- asking how patients have coped and are coping.
- introducing new skills to broaden a patient's repertoire (behavioral, cognitive, emotional, existential).

COLLABORATING WITH COLLEAGUES

Our coping support is not limited to patients and families. Oncologists report difficult challenges when caring for patients with incurable cancer, including emotionally draining communication, responsibility for life and death, and the limitations of oncology to heal. Because our palliative care workroom is situated inside the cancer center, sharing space and services, and because we are in touch frequently, oncologists know that we are near at hand when they need support. Even with virtual care, we have tried to replicate this environment by continuing to have one in-person clinician stationed in our workroom. Our oncology colleagues freely reach out to get curbside advice, make urgent referrals, and talk through a difficult case. We support our oncologists with empathic listening and humor and by partnering with them on difficult cases. As one oncology colleague told us, "I feel the most supported when the palliative care clinician joins me in the deep end of the pool."

MEETING THE CHALLENGE OF LIVING WELL
WITH SERIOUS ILLNESS

In this chapter, we have discussed how to use times of stability to help patients live well with serious illness. The challenge of living well presents itself throughout the illness. Patients may meet this challenge to varying degrees on different days or in different moments on any single day. We empathize with this difficulty and provide ongoing encouragement and coaching.

For those patients initially unable to pair hope and worries, the focus on living well can build increased coping capacity that allows them to acknowledge worries. For these patients, we might move back and forth between the third and second challenges. To begin, we first ask patients to consider how to live well even though they are facing serious illness.

Then we help patients reinforce and develop a wide range of coping skills.

Living well with the illness is a central goal of early integrated palliative care, and clinicians should spend the most time on this challenge. Patients who take it up report better outcomes. They feel more like their old self. Sometimes they even forget about having cancer. Once patients have times when they live well with their cancer, we can move to the fourth challenge: deepening prognostic awareness. The decision to move on will depend on the patient's desire to think ahead and on the pace of the illness. The following schema shows patients' motion through and among the challenges.

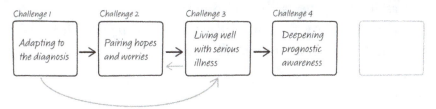

COMMUNICATION SKILLS SUMMARY

CHAPTER 1: ADAPTING TO THE DIAGNOSIS

Assess prognostic awareness: What is your understanding of your illness? Looking to the future, what are your hopes? What are your worries?

Support coping: Normalize, align, contain.

Be an interpreter: Interpret the patient for the oncologist and the oncologist for the patient.

CHAPTER 2: PAIRING HOPES AND WORRIES

For patients who focus solely on hope: Align with hope and touch upon the illness by

- empathizing
- understanding the illness's impact on others

- suggesting a worried part
- mentioning the "what ifs"
- linking to worries with "even though"

For patients who acknowledge hopes and worries: Pair the patient's hopes and worries, and normalize these mixed feelings.

CHAPTER 3: LIVING WELL WITH SERIOUS ILLNESS
Promote healthy coping by
- exploring what it means to live well with the illness
- asking how patients have coped and are coping
- introducing new skills to broaden the patient's repertoire (behavioral, cognitive, emotional, existential)

FURTHER READING

Arean, P., Hegel, M., Vannoy, S., Fan, M. Y, & Unuzter, J. (2008). Effectiveness of problem-solving therapy for older, primary care patients with depression: Results from the Impact Project. *Gerontologist, 48*(3), 311–323.

Bluhm, M., Connell, C. M., De Vries, R. G., Janz, N. K., Bickel, K. E., & Silveira, M. J. (2016). Paradox of prescribing late chemotherapy: Oncologists explain. *Journal of Oncology Practice, 12*(12), e1006–e1015.

Breitbart, W., Pessin, H., Rosenfeld, B., Applebaum, A. J., Lichtenthal, W. G., Li, Y., Saracino, R. M., Marziliano, A. M., Masterson, M., Tobias, K., & Fenn, N. (2018). Individual meaning-centered psychotherapy for the treatment of psychological and existential distress: A randomized controlled trial in patients with advanced cancer. *Cancer, 124*(15), 3231–3239.

Chirico, A., Lucidi, F., Merluzzi, T., Alivernini, F., Laurentiis, M., Botti, G., & Giordano, A. (2017). A meta-analytic review of the relationship of cancer coping self-efficacy with distress and quality of life. *Oncotarget, 8*(22), 36800–36811.

Chirico, A., Serpentini, S., Merluzzi, T., Mallia, L., Del Bianco, P., Martino, R., Trentin, L., Bucci, E., De Laurentiis, M., Capovilla, E., Lucidi, F., Botti, G., & Giordano, A. (2017). Self-efficacy for coping moderates the effects of distress on quality of life in palliative cancer care. *Anticancer Research, 37*(4), 1609–1615.

Delgado-Guay, M. O., Parsons, H. A., Hui, D., De la Cruz, M. G., Thorney, S., & Bruera, E. (2013). Spirituality, religiosity, and spiritual pain among caregivers of patients with advanced cancer. *American Journal of Hospice and Palliative Care, 30*(5), 455–461.

Fitchett, G., Emanuel, L., Handzo, G., Boyken, L., & Wilkie, D. J. (2015). Care of the human spirit and the role of dignity therapy: A systematic review of dignity therapy research. *BMC Palliative Care, 14*, 8.

Folkman, S., & Lazarus, R. S. (1988). The relationship between coping and emotion: Implications for theory and research. *Social Science and Medicine, 26*(3), 309–317.

Fredrickson, B. L. (2001). The role of positive emotions in positive psychology: The broaden-and-build theory of positive emotions. *American Psychologist, 56*(3), 218–226.

Greer, J. A., Applebaum, A. J., Jacobsen, J. C., Temel, J. S., & Jackson, V. A. (2020). Understanding and addressing the role of coping in palliative care for patients with advanced cancer. *Journal of Clinical Oncology, 38*(9), 915–925.

Greer, J. A., Jacobs, J. M., El-Jawahri, A., Nipp, R. D., Gallagher, E. R., Pirl, W. F., Park, E. R., Muzikansky, A., Jacobsen, J. C., Jackson, V. A., & Temel, J. S. (2018). Role of patient coping strategies in understanding the effects of early palliative care on quality of life and mood. *Journal of Clinical Oncology, 36*(1), 53–60.

Heckhausen, J., Wrosch, C., & Schulz, R. (2010). A motivational theory of life-span development. *Psychological Review, 117*(1), 32–60.

Hirai, K., Motooka, H., Ito, N., Wada, N., Yoshizaki, A., Shiozaki, M., Momino, K., Okuyama, T., & Akechi, T. (2012). Problem-solving therapy for psychological distress in Japanese early-stage breast cancer patients. *Japanese Journal of Clinical Oncology, 42*(12), 1168–1174.

Hoerger, M., Greer, J. A., Jackson, V. A., Park, E. R., Pirl, W. F., El-Jawahri, A., Gallagher, E. R., Hagan, T., Jacobsen, J., Perry, L. M., & Temel, J. S. (2018). Defining the elements of early palliative care that are associated with patient-reported outcomes and the delivery of end-of-life care. *Journal of Clinical Oncology, 36*(11), 1096–1102.

Jacobsen, J., Kvale, E., Rabow, M., Rinaldi, S., Cohen, S., Weissman, E., & Jackson, V. (2014). Helping patients with serious illness live well through the promotion of adaptive coping: A report from the Improving Outpatient Palliative Care (IPAL-OP) initiative. *Journal of Palliative Medicine, 17*(4), 463–468.

Kobau, R., Seligman, M. E., Peterson, C., Diener, E., Zack, M. M., Chapman, E., & Thompson, W. (2011). Mental health promotion in public health: Perspectives and strategies from positive psychology. *American Journal of Public Health, 101*(8), e1–e9.

Lazarus, R. S., & Folkman, S. (1984). *Stress, appraisal, and coping.* Springer.

Maciejewski, P. K., Phelps, A. C., Kacel, E. L., Balboni, T. A., Balboni, M., Wright, A. A., Pirl, W., & Prigerson, H. G. (2012). Religious coping and behavioral disengagement: Opposing influences on advance care planning and receipt of intensive care near death. *Psycho-Oncology, 21*(7), 714–723.

Morris, N., Moghaddam, N., Tickle, A., & Biswas, S. (2018). The relationship between coping style and psychological distress in people with head and neck cancer: A systematic review. *Psycho-Oncology, 27*(3), 734–747.

Nezu, A., Nezu, C., Friedman, S., Faddis, S., & Houts, P. (1999). *Helping cancer patients cope: A problem-solving approach.* American Psychological Association.

Nipp, R. D., El-Jawahri, A., Fishbein, J. N., Eusebio, J., Stagl, J. M., Gallagher, E. R., Park, E. R., Jackson, V. A., Pirl, W. F., Greer, J. A., & Temel, J. S. (2016). The relationship between coping strategies, quality of life, and mood in patients with incurable cancer. *Cancer, 122*(13), 2110–2116.

Nipp, R., Greer, J., El-Jawahri, A., Moran, S., Traeger, L., Jacobs, J., Jacobsen, J., Gallagher, E. R., Park, E. R., Ryan, D. P., Jackson, V. A., Pirl, W. F., & Temel, J. S. (2017). Coping and prognostic awareness in patients with advanced cancer. *Journal of Clinical Oncology, 35*(22), 2551–2557.

Panagioti, M., Gooding, P. A., & Tarrier, N. (2012). An empirical investigation of the effectiveness of the broad-minded affective coping procedure (BMAC) to boost mood among individuals with posttraumatic stress disorder (PTSD). *Behaviour Research and Therapy, 50*(10), 589–595.

Phelps, A. C., Maciejewski, P. K., Nilsson, M., Balboni, T. A., Wright, A. A., Paulk, M. E., Trice, E., Schrag, D., Peteet, J. R., Block, S. D., & Prigerson, H. G. (2009). Religious coping and use of intensive life-prolonging care near death in patients with advanced cancer. *Journal of the American Medical Association, 301*(11), 1140–1147.

Pierce, D. (2012). Problem solving therapy: Use and effectiveness in general practice. *Australian Family Physician, 41*(9), 676–679.

Puchalski, C. M. (2014). The FICA Spiritual History Tool #274. *Journal of Palliative Medicine, 17*(1), 105–106.

Rand, K. L., Cripe, L. D., Monahan, P. O., Tong, Y., Schmidt, K., & Rawl, S. M. (2012). Illness appraisal, religious coping, and psychological responses in men with advanced cancer. *Supportive Care in Cancer, 20*(8), 1719–1728.

Salsman, J. M., Pustejovsky, J. E., Jim, H. S., Munoz, A. R., Merluzzi, T. V., George, L., Park, C. L., Danhauer, S. C., Sherman, A. C., Snyder, M. A., & Fitchett, G. (2015). A meta-analytic approach to examining the correlation between religion/spirituality and mental health in cancer. *Cancer, 121*(21), 3769–3778.

Schreuders, B., van Oppen, P., van Marwijk, H. W., Smit, J. H., & Stalman, W. A. (2005). Frequent attenders in general practice: Problem solving treatment provided by nurses. *BMC Family Practice, 6*, 42.

Skinner, E. A., Edge, K., Altman, J., & Sherwood, H. (2003). Searching for the structure of coping: A review and critique of category systems for classifying ways of coping. *Psychological Bulletin, 129*(2), 216–269.

Tarakeshwar, N., Vanderwerker, L. C., Paulk, E., Pearce, M. J., Kasl, S. V., & Prigerson, H. G. (2006). Religious coping is associated with the quality of life of patients with advanced cancer. *Journal of Palliative Medicine, 9*(3), 646–657.

Trevino, K. M., Balboni, M., Zollfrank, A., Balboni, T., & Prigerson, H. G. (2014). Negative religious coping as a correlate of suicidal ideation in patients with advanced cancer. *Psycho-Oncology, 23*(8), 936–945.

True, G., Phipps, E. J., Braitman, L. E., Harralson, T., Harris, D., & Tester, W. (2005). Treatment preferences and advance care planning at end of life: The role of ethnicity and spiritual coping in cancer patients. *Annals of Behavioral Medicine, 30*(2), 174–179.

Vallurupalli, M., Lauderdale, K., Balboni, M. J., Phelps, A. C., Block, S. D., Ng, A. K., Kachnic, L. A., Vanderweele, T. J., & Balboni, T. A. (2012). The role of spirituality and religious coping in the quality of life of patients with advanced cancer receiving palliative radiation therapy. *Journal of Supportive Oncology,* *10*(2), 81–87.

Winkelman, W. D., Lauderdale, K., Balboni, M. J., Phelps, A. C., Peteet, J. R., Block, S. D., Kachnic, L. A., VanderWeele, T. J., & Balboni, T. A. (2011). The relationship of spiritual concerns to the quality of life of advanced cancer patients: Preliminary findings. *Journal of Palliative Medicine, 14*(9), 1022–1028.

Deepening Prognostic Awareness

Sonya, a patient in her 40s with advanced pancreatic cancer, has been working with palliative care during the 6 months since her diagnosis. She met the first challenge of adapting to her diagnosis and agreed to palliative care helping her live well even though she faces cancer, the clinician's pairing of hopes and worries.

Yet Sonya struggles to talk in any detail about her worries, particularly since moving to second-line treatment. She copes by focusing on optimistic hope and avoiding negative thoughts. Her other main coping mechanism is the distraction of work. She maintains the accounts for her brother's automotive repair shop. She says that project keeps her mind off the cancer. Six months after diagnosis, she still asks that her palliative care visits focus on being positive because any negative thinking would weaken her immune system.

THE CHALLENGE OF DEEPENING PROGNOSTIC AWARENESS

Sonya's clinician is not sure how he can help. Despite Sonya working with him for many months, she acknowledges worries only briefly and quickly signals that she is not ready to talk more. Yet, as her clinician knows, Sonya's progression to second-line treatment means that her prognosis is short, likely 6 months or less, and he wants her to consider this possibility.

Doing so would help Sonya choose how to spend her time and help her prepare for end-of-life decisions. In short, Sonya needs help taking up the fourth challenge: deepening prognostic awareness.

Sonya uses distraction and optimistic hope to keep her worries at a distance. But even patients who can more readily acknowledge worries need help thinking about the future. When patients initially pair hopes and worries, taking up the second challenge, they might simply hear the clinician's pairing. Or they might name an inchoate worry, such as acknowledging the illness is "not good" or that they are upset. This level of generality makes planning difficult. Thus, in this fourth challenge, we invite patients to talk more explicitly about worries, to reflect on the meaning of the prognosis—on how the illness is changing their lives. They might be asked how they would like to spend their remaining time, if time were short. As patients consider the meaning of the prognosis, inchoate worries become more detailed, a process represented by the worried circle expanding (Figure 4.1). These conversations prepare patients emotionally

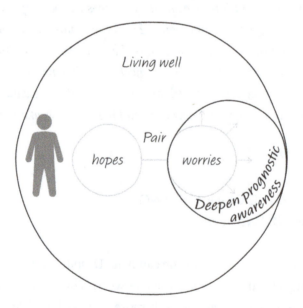

Figure 4.1 Adding challenge 4: deepening prognostic awareness. As patients consider the meaning of the prognosis, inchoate worries become more detailed, a process represented by the expanding worries circle.

for when their bodies signal that the cancer is progressing, when treatment won't be effective. They can even help patients move toward acceptance.

The necessary tasks of talking about the future and deepening prognostic awareness are distressing. *Distress tolerance* describes the capacity to experience oneself and the current challenging situation without trying to change the situation. Building distress tolerance (which begins when we introduce palliative care) is an extensively researched therapeutic approach. It is an important component of dialectical behavioral therapy (DBT), a cognitive-behavioral therapy centered on the dialectic of acceptance and change that teaches patients skills to cope with highly emotional situations. In DBT, patients learn distress tolerance skills to get through a crisis (including crises caused by addictive behaviors). But distress tolerance helps all patients under stress. For patients facing serious illness, we build distress tolerance by inviting, but not forcing, them to talk about the future and supporting them emotionally through these conversations.

This chapter discusses how. We discuss approaches for the many patients who can already talk about the future (who more easily pair hopes and worries). Then we focus on the patients most needing specialist palliative care: patients like Sonya, who are hesitant to talk about getting sicker even as their illness progresses. We show how to invite patients who are hesitant into these difficult conversations and discuss how clinical attunement can help. Finally, we discuss how shifts in patients' prognostic awareness can impact collaboration with colleagues.

HOW TO HELP PATIENTS DEEPEN
PROGNOSTIC AWARENESS

Patients more easily accept our invitations to conversations that deepen prognostic awareness after they have met the third challenge, living well with serious illness. Our focus on living well builds trust and teaches coping skills. With some patients, we touch upon worries initially with the second challenge, spend months on living well, and then move to deepening prognostic awareness. With other patients, we move back and forth between living well and deepening prognostic awareness within one visit. The frequent returns to living well give patients needed breaks from the intensity of the prognosis.

In either case, we still begin each visit by building rapport and confirming that symptoms are managed. If the patient is experiencing physical distress, we defer our conversation about deepening prognostic awareness to another day. Otherwise, our next step is to assess the patient's prognostic awareness on that day (we say "on that day" because prognostic awareness changes from day to day and even minute to minute). If the patient can acknowledge worries, we usually begin the conversation. But we first note what else is going on in the patient's life. If an important event, perhaps a birthday or trip, is coming up, we would wait so that the conversation does not overshadow the event. We would also wait if the patient has specific worries unrelated to the illness. For example, if a patient moving to a different home is focused on the myriad details of the move, we might instead problem solve how to ask for social support.

When we begin a conversation to deepen prognostic awareness, we try to calibrate our language to the patient's readiness for distressing topics. Words, like medications, have different potencies. Here is a gentle (1-mg strength) question: "Do you let yourself think about the 'what ifs' with this cancer?" This question merely alludes to distressing situations. A stronger (10-mg strength) question might be, "Do you let yourself think about the possibility of getting sicker?" This question is more specific to the illness. A direct (100-mg strength) question might be, "Do you let yourself think about the possibility of dying from this cancer?" We start gently and judge increases in potency by hearing and reflecting the patient's language.

Conversations to deepen prognostic awareness can include information about how much time remains (even roughly) or what that time might be like, especially when patients ask. But conversations to deepen prognostic awareness range beyond, and need not include, explicit prognostic disclosures. They instead focus on the general idea that time is shorter than hoped and help patients understand what this idea means for them. This less explicit framing is often all that is needed to deepen prognostic awareness.

Patients Who Can Talk about the Future

Patients who can pair hopes and worries have some distress tolerance and can begin a more explicit conversation about the future. We help them to increase distress tolerance and deepen prognostic awareness by using the generalist advance care planning approaches of serious illness conversations and advance directives.

SERIOUS ILLNESS CONVERSATIONS

Serious illness conversations are a generalist approach to building distress tolerance and deepening prognostic awareness. Even when patients can talk about the future, many do not realize that serious illness conversations range beyond the very end of life and include themes that will improve quality of life throughout the illness.

These conversations help patients cope. They are associated with reductions in patients' anxiety and depression. Furthermore, when patients understand how their time or function may be limited as the illness progresses, they often change their goals: "I think I'll take that trip this summer." They cope better also because they understand that we will talk with them about end of life when necessary. As one patient said, "I know that you will let me know when things are going south, so I mostly try to forget about all of this."

Ariadne Labs in Boston has created a "Serious Illness Conversation Guide," listing questions to facilitate these conversations. (Clinicians are encouraged to hold and follow the guide as they talk with patients.) For our clinical work at Massachusetts General Hospital, we adopted and adapted the Serious Illness Conversation Guide (licensed under a Creative Commons ShareAlike license that encourages reuse and adaptation). Our guide begins with a conversation opener and then turns to an assessment of the patient's prognostic awareness (Box 4.1). This assessment helps us to decide whether today is right for a conversation and to base our conversation on the patient's current hopes and worries. In the third section of the guide, "Share Worry," the clinician aligns with the patient's hopes and pairs them with a prognostic disclosure. Even patients who can acknowledge worries take in prognostic information more easily when worries are paired with hope.

Box 4.1 SERIOUS ILLNESS CONVERSATION GUIDE

OPEN THE CONVERSATION

I'd like to talk about what is ahead with your illness. Would that be okay?

ASSESS PROGNOSTIC AWARENESS

What is your **understanding** of your illness?

Looking to the future, what are your **hopes** about your health?

What are your **worries**?

SHARE WORRY

Would it be okay if we talked more about what may lie ahead?

FUNCTION: I **hear** you're hoping for _____ and I **worry** the decline we have seen is going to continue.

TIME: I **hear** you're hoping for _____ and I **worry** something serious may happen in the next few (weeks/months/years).

ALIGN

I **wish** we didn't have to worry about this.

EXPLORE WHAT'S IMPORTANT

If your health situation worsens, what is **most important** to you?

How much do your **family or friends** know about your priorities and wishes?

MAKE A RECOMMENDATION

It sounds like _____ is very important to you.

Given what's important to you, **I recommend . . .**

DOCUMENT YOUR CONVERSATION

This material has been modified by us. Original content @ https://portal.ariadnelabs.org licensed under CC-BY-SA-4.0 by Ariadne Labs.

Questions about a patient's hopes, worries, and what matters most open a wide range of conversations covering many themes including:

- the impact of the illness on the patient's goals for the time remaining, leading to new or revised goals;
- the impact of the illness on the patient's roles at home, at work, or in the community, leading to reimagining how to spend time;
- the impact of the illness on loved ones, leading to ways of helping them;
- physical suffering, leading to ways that clinicians can help manage symptoms;
- anticipatory grief, including spiritual and emotional suffering, leading to ways that these hardships can be eased;
- the patient's experiences and legacy, leading to ways of finding meaning and purpose;
- the logistics of dying, leading to ways of finding the right support;
- values and priorities at the end of life related to medical care, leading to a care plan;
- information preferences, leading to more attuned conversations about the illness and prognosis.

Some themes may have been explored for the third challenge in conversations about living well, which needed only implicit acknowledgment of the prognosis. Now, as the prognosis becomes more definite and the patient's understanding of it more explicit, these themes can be revisited with more specificity. In the following example, the patient asks for guidance on thinking about how much to know. The example illustrates that these conversations need not involve an explicit prognostic disclosure.

Working with a patient to deepen prognostic awareness

DIALOG	OUR PERSPECTIVE
PATIENT: I can't even believe this is happening. How do I even think about it?	

DIALOG	OUR PERSPECTIVE
CLINICIAN: In terms of knowing prognostic information, some people find it helpful to get our best sense of it. Other people say, "That wouldn't be helpful to me at all." And sometimes people say, as you do, "I don't really think this is happening . . . I've got all the information. But in my head, I'm not there yet." At some point, it can be helpful to imagine, "What if I were very sick? I don't feel like I am now. But if I were, here is my sense of how I would want this to go."	*Explains how patients have different preferences for prognostic information, implying that the patient does not have to have an explicit discussion. Then, suggests that at some point it would be helpful to think ahead and plan for end of life.*
PATIENT: Yep. So probably a good half step, which makes sense to me, would be for me to at least write down for myself.	*Considers how he might begin to think about end of life.*
CLINICIAN: Right, to do your own sort of work. I think that makes perfect sense.	*Supports the idea that thinking about the future is the patient's task.*
PATIENT: Yeah. Because there are things that I would want and other things that I may need to talk to you more thoroughly about.	*Reflects more.*
CLINICIAN: Yeah. That's why this is a process.	*Reframes this reflection as a process.*

DIALOG	OUR PERSPECTIVE
PATIENT: Mm-hmm. It's a process.	
CLINICIAN: It's not like we flip a switch. Some people are pretty clear about it, but for the vast majority it's a process.	*Normalizes the process.*
PATIENT: Yeah, well, if I were 80 . . .	
CLINICIAN: (laughter) It's still a process.	

Over time, as patients trust us and understand that these conversations are a process, they talk more about their worries. One patient with incurable lung cancer initially spoke about the illness's effect on her adult children. Only after months of working with her did she mention her sadness and longing for her elderly parents, unable to visit due to pandemic-related restrictions.

As Ariadne Lab's Serious Illness Care Program spreads, serious illness conversations will be increasingly conducted by nonpalliative care specialists and documented in the electronic medical record. In our hospital system, serious illness conversations are often held and documented by oncology colleagues, giving the whole team a base from which to deepen patients' prognostic awareness.

We do so by first asking about previous serious illness conversations: "Has your oncologist had a conversation with you about the big picture?" We ask this regardless of whether a conversation is documented in the medical record.

If patients answer no, we ask whether it would be helpful to think ahead: "Patients have big picture conversations with their oncologist. These conversations are also part of our job as palliative care clinicians. Would it be helpful to take a step back and think about what lies ahead with your illness?"

If patients answer yes, we ask follow-up questions inviting patients to reflect on what they learned from the conversation and on how that information affects them. Here are typical follow-up questions:

- "What was the conversation like?"
- "What did you learn?"
- "How did the conversation change your perspective on how you live?"
- "What are you hoping for now?"
- "What are your biggest worries now?"
- "What are your priorities now?"

ADVANCE DIRECTIVES

Although the focus of advance care planning has shifted from completing advance directive documents to conducting serious illness conversations, clinicians can still deepen patients' prognostic awareness by filling out the forms (either on paper or electronically). These forms include the health care proxy form or more specific advance directives such as the Medical Orders for Life-Sustaining Treatment (MOLST). They can be filled out by primary care clinicians, but completion rates are low, whether for patients with chronic disease (38.2%) or for healthy adults (32.7%). Thus, we need to encourage completion. Our research showed that palliative care clinicians tend to complete advance directives with patients in the last few visits of life (Figure 1.2). This delay represents a missed opportunity because completing these forms—especially the health care proxy—is an easy way to invite patients to consider the meaning of the prognosis.

Health care proxy completion is safe to ask about. Because the form is universal (the form is standard), procedural (it's a form), and hypothetical (patients might never need the proxy), its completion does not evoke strong feelings. The clinician might simply ask, "Have you chosen somebody to be your medical decision maker in the event of an emergency? It is important that everyone has one." The language normalizes the process, as most patients agree on the importance of planning for an emergency that could happen to everyone.

When patients are open to completing the form, we invite them to a deeper conversation: "One part of choosing a medical decision maker is completing the form. The second part is a conversation with your medical decision maker about your priorities if your health were to worsen. Have you started that kind of conversation?"

For many patients, this depth of conversation is tolerable. However, it can be too much for some. Sonya, our patient at the start of the chapter with advanced pancreatic cancer, simply deferred the conversation, saying, "I don't want to think about that right now." We don't push patients like Sonya to continue the conversation or even to choose a medical decision maker. By asking the question, we have already helped her build distress tolerance.

Another procedural invitation to consider the future is the MOLST form. But we don't simply ask, "Do you want CPR?" Instead, we recommend care based on the patient's goals and values and on the medical situation. Thus, early in the illness, we often recommend CPR: "Given that you are strong and still working and that your goal is to live as long as possible, I would recommend CPR if you should have a sudden emergency."

As the illness progresses and CPR offers less benefit, we talk about it again. (Our first conversation has built distress tolerance for the next.) We tell patients of our growing concern that, as the cancer spreads, CPR becomes less likely to help them live longer or better, and we frequently recommend a do-not-resuscitate (DNR) order: "I know that you have worried about suffering and that you want things to be peaceful at the end. I too am worried. I am getting worried that the risks of suffering with CPR may outweigh the benefits. I would recommend that, in a medical emergency, we focus on your comfort and not do CPR."

Many patients do not at first take our recommendation and remain full code. A difficult transition takes time. Thus, we begin these "I'm worried" conversations early, when patients start to decline. If a patient wants to remain full code, we do not complete the MOLST form. A full-code MOLST form is superfluous and, when the patient declines to where CPR is very unlikely to be beneficial, can even burden the family's decision-making.

When patients getting sicker want to remain full code, we mention subsequent conversations. We explain that, if we become very worried that aggressive treatments like CPR would cause harm, we will revisit the topic. We also explain that CPR will eventually not be medically indicated because it cannot halt the dying process. We reassure our patients that, when that time comes, we will let them know. Mentioning these turning points prompts the patient to think ahead, thereby building distress tolerance for our next conversation. In the following dialog, the palliative care clinician and the oncologist explain to a patient how the recommendation process might work.

Foreshadowing a recommendation

PALLIATIVE CARE CLINICIAN: You know, Dr. [oncologist] and I, in these situations, often make recommendations to people. We'll say, we think that this option makes sense, we think this intervention doesn't make sense.

ONCOLOGIST: And I think it will be pretty clear-cut. If we're doing heroic measures, and we get to the point that they won't help, Dr. [palliative care clinician] and I, and whatever team is taking care of you, would know when we're at that point. We would recommend to you and your family that we stop what we're doing.

Patients Hesitant to Discuss the Future

Patients hesitant to discuss the future can hear our pairing and may acknowledge worries briefly, but cannot discuss them explicitly. The clinician's the natural temptation is to avoid these explicit conversations. However, in addition to helping patients cope, these conversations, and little else, prepare patients for shared decision-making. Thus, we consider whether these benefits make the patient's momentary distress worth tolerating (by us and the patient). The answer might change from day to day depending on the patient's coping and the pace of the illness progression. We also remind ourselves that the patient's distress is caused by the diagnosis and is present before any conversation that we invite.

To approach distressing conversations without overwhelming patients requires clinical attunement (introduced in Chapter 2): a responsiveness to the patient's needs that takes into account how the patient is coping and the mostly likely illness trajectory. Clinical attunement helps any patient deepen prognostic awareness but is particularly important with patients who are hesitant. These patients, leery of talking about the future, cue us often to change the topic. Because we encourage the conversation despite their cues, we must be particularly gentle to help the patient modulate the conversation's emotional intensity. The following sections discuss skills for staying attuned to the patient's needs at the beginning, throughout, and at the close of a conversation (Figure 4.2).

Beginning a Conversation

To start a conversation with a patient who is hesitant, we can align with hope by repeating back the patient's hopes using his or her words. This alignment builds rapport and communicates that all emotions are welcome. (Patients sometimes mistakenly assume that palliative care is only about dying.) Alternatively, we can acknowledge hope: We recognize the hopeful feeling without aligning fully with the specific hope. There are

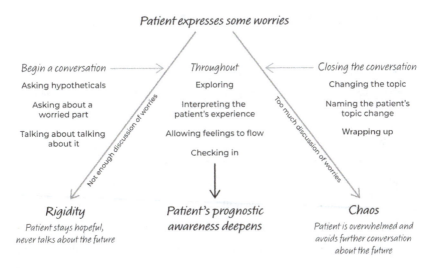

Figure 4.2 Skills for clinical attunement at the beginning, throughout, and at the close of a conversation

two ways. The first is to repeat back the patient's hope and add our more achievable hope of helping the patient live well: "I know that you are 100% focused on beating this cancer. My hope is that together we can help you live well." (This combination is a subtle pairing of hope and worry, with the worry implicit in the difference between the patient's hope and our addition.) The second way to acknowledge hope (also implicitly pairing hope and worry) is to name a related, more achievable hope—for example, to the patient 100% focused on beating the cancer: "I know that you are hoping to fight this cancer" (Table 4.1).

With patients who express a range of hopes, optimistic and achievable, we can choose aligning or acknowledging. However, with patients who are very optimistically hopeful, we align. These patients need the hopes to cope. We may emphasize our alignment by looking at the patient directly when we repeat back hopes and by speaking clearly and slowly. Only once these patients see and hear that we understand their hopes can they consider talking more about worries.

With patients who are hesitant, to begin talking about worries we use three approaches: hypothetical questions, the worried part, and talk about talking about it.

Table 4.1 Working with the Hope "I Am 100% Focused on Beating This Cancer"

Aligning with the patient's hope	
Reflecting back	"I know that you are 100% focused on beating this cancer."
Acknowledging hope	
Adding to the patient's hope	"I know that you are 100% focused on beating this cancer. My hope is that together we can help you live well."
Naming a related, more achievable hope	"I know that you are hoping to fight this cancer."
	"I know that you are hoping to control this cancer and live a long time."
	"I know that you are hoping to live well as possible."

Hypothetical Questions

Hypothetical questions are a safe beginning because they imply that the outcome is uncertain and offer psychological distance from it. (In the following examples, the clinician's alignment with hope is bolded and the hypothetical question, an analog for worry, is italicized.)

- **"I am hoping with you that this chemotherapy controls the cancer for a long time.** *I also wonder, if it were to stop working at some point, what would be your most important priorities?"*
- **"I hear you are hoping to live as well as possible.** *Part of my job is to help people prepare for the 'what ifs.' If time were getting short, how would you want to spend that time?"*

Because the future is "ever in motion" (Yoda), this indirect approach has truth and integrity early in the illness. (A more direct approach is required when the questions are no longer hypothetical—for example, when chemotherapy is no longer working. This situation is discussed in Chapter 5.)

A still safer hypothetical question leaves the outcome undefined: "I know that you are focused on fighting this illness. And I wonder, do you ever let yourself think about the 'what ifs'?" The patient can then identify which "what if" to discuss. It might be a specific short-term concern, such as the treatment being delayed or the dose reduced, or an existential topic.

Every hypothetical question should be asked with care, as even hypothetical possibilities can be frightening. A patient becoming overwhelmed might change the subject or give nonverbal cues like looking down, crossing arms and legs, or leaving the room in search of water or the bathroom. If the conversation seems to be getting overwhelming, we check: "Is it okay for us to be talking about this?" If needed, we'll halt the conversation and try another day.

In the following example, the clinician brings up a "what if" with Sonya, who is stable on second-line chemotherapy and hesitant to talk about the future.

Working with Sonya using a hypothetical approach ("what ifs")

DIALOG	OUR PERSPECTIVE
CLINICIAN: I came to check in and see how things are going with you.	
SONYA: Well, doing the best I can. Fighting. I need to stay strong in this.	
CLINICIAN: Of course. You doing okay with the chemotherapy? Symptoms under control?	
SONYA: Best I can. I'm not going to complain. Scans looked good last month.	
CLINICIAN: I am so glad that you are doing well and that the cancer is controlled. You and I have worked hard on your symptoms, so that you can feel well and so that you can fight this. Now that we are in this stable time, part of my job is also to think through with you a little bit about the "what ifs."	*Aligns with hopes to live well and fight and touches upon worries using the "what ifs" (framing them as a role of the palliative care clinician).*
SONYA: What does that mean?	
CLINICIAN: For all my patients, I have found that it can be helpful to consider what might be ahead. For example, if these treatments should stop controlling the cancer, what might be your most important goals?	*Asks a hypothetical "what if" question.*

DIALOG	OUR PERSPECTIVE
SONYA: Well, I obviously want it to work. Sometimes I worry about if it didn't, what would they come up with next? I mean, I think that they would come up with something else, a different way to attack it, from a different angle. Because I'm not the type of person that just gives up.	*Focuses on hopes.*
CLINICIAN: It is hard to live with so much uncertainty. I also hear that it is important for you to keep looking at options and thinking about treatments.	*Pairs worries with hopes: empathizes with the illness experience of uncertainty (the worry) and aligns with Sonya's hope for more treatments if needed.*
SONYA: Oh yeah, absolutely.	

Sonya does not want to discuss what happens if the treatments run out. Sensing Sonya's hesitance, the clinician does not push her—and need not, for he has already gently invited Sonya to consider the meaning of the prognosis simply by asking the hypothetical question. These gentle invitations gradually build Sonya's distress tolerance.

The Worried Part

A second and gentler way to invite patients to consider the meaning of the prognosis is to ask about a worried part: "I hear you are hoping to beat this. Is there also a part of you that worries about what might lie ahead?" Many patients can acknowledge at least a worried *part*, finding worries more manageable when seen as smaller or partial.

In the following illustrative dialog, Sonya's clinician asks a "parts" question. The example begins with the same dialog as the preceding example and diverges from it at the parts question.

Working with Sonya using a parts question

DIALOG	OUR PERSPECTIVE
CLINICIAN: I came to check in and see how things are going with you.	
SONYA: Well, doing the best I can. Fighting. I need to stay strong in this.	
CLINICIAN: Of course. You doing okay with the chemotherapy? Symptoms under control?	
SONYA: Best I can. I'm not going to complain. Scans looked good last month.	*Acknowledges excellent symptom control (including pain).*
CLINICIAN: I am so glad that you are doing well and that the cancer is controlled. You and I have worked hard on your symptoms, so that you can feel well and fight this. The part of you that fights this illness is strong! I wonder, as you face all of this, is there also a part of you that worries about what lies ahead?	*Aligns with hopes and asks indirectly about the future using a "parts" approach.*
SONYA: Of course! But it's just so hard to think about.	*Does not reject outright the gentle parts-focused invitation: Talking about it is hard but not too hard.*
CLINICIAN: Can you tell me more?	
SONYA: I just worry that I am not going to feel strong again, that this is going to keep going.	*Sonya can talk about her fears.*

Dialog	Our perspective
CLINICIAN: Yes, cancer is scary.	*Expresses empathy by naming the emotion.*
SONYA: I wonder if I should start back on the OxyContin. Sometimes I think that pain block might be fading a little. They said it would in a few months.	*Changes topic to symptoms (just acknowledged as well controlled), indicating that she cannot think more about the future right then.*
CLINICIAN: It sounds like, for today, it would be more helpful to talk about your pain rather than to think more generally about the future. Is that right?	*Acknowledges the topic change and suggests that they might talk about the future on a different day.*

Patients, like Sonya, who are still hesitant even after a parts approach need the gentlest approach, discussed next. (Patients who exhibit this persistent one-sidedness, focusing exclusively on hopes, should also be screened and treated for depression and may benefit from psychiatric referral.)

Talking About Talking About It

The third and gentlest approach to begin a conversation about worries involves not talking about the future directly but instead "talking about talking about it [the future]." The agenda items of this meta-conversation include the logistics of a conversation about the future, the advantages and disadvantages of a conversation, and the patient's information preferences.

Exploring the logistics of the proposed conversation helps patients consider a conversation about the future from a safe distance. A logistics conversation requires neither discussion of the illness nor a medical decision. Its agenda includes whom to include in a conversation about the future and when and where to hold it. It can also include the advantages and disadvantages of a conversation about the future, which helps patients recognize their fears and acknowledge benefits to the conversation. Articulating fears and benefits can change them from vague feelings into reasons that can be evaluated and weighed against each other.

Table 4.2 QUESTIONS FOR "TALKING ABOUT TALKING ABOUT IT"

Discussing logistics	"If we were going to have a conversation, whom should we include?"
	"Where might we hold this conversation?"
	"How might we know when it is the right time?"
Considering pros and cons	"What might be some advantages of holding a conversation about the future?"
	"Can you tell me about disadvantages?"
	"Could we overcome those disadvantages?"

Table 4.2 lists questions for talking about talking about it. Patients who are the most hesitant might tolerate only one or two questions per visit and need several months talking about the conversation before holding it.

Here is an example conversation illustrating "talking about talking about it," continuing after Sonya switches the topic to symptoms.

Trying "Talk about talking about it"

DIALOG	OUR PERSPECTIVE
CLINICIAN: It sounds like, for today, it would be more helpful to talk about your pain rather than to think more generally about the future. Is that right?	*Acknowledges the topic change and suggests that they might talk about the future on a different day.*
SONYA: I just want to focus on good things for now.	
CLINICIAN: I know that it is important for you to be positive. Let's definitely return to pain control. Before we do that, can you share a little about what you see as the biggest disadvantages of talking about the future?	*Aligns with hope and change of topic before exploring the disadvantages of a conversation.*

Dialog	Our perspective
SONYA: It is just so overwhelming. I just can't do it.	
CLINICIAN: I hear that. And we certainly do not have to have that conversation today. Though I wonder, might there be any advantages in talking a bit about the future at another visit?	*Aligns with the wish not to talk about the future on that day and explores possible advantages.*
SONYA: Well, it is good to be prepared. I can see that.	*Acknowledges an advantage.*
CLINICIAN: It can be helpful for people to think ahead and make plans. Maybe next time we can think together to plan that conversation. It would be helpful to know whom to include.	*Mentions a second "talking about talking about it" conversation.*
SONYA: I will think about that.	
CLINICIAN: Let's talk about this more next time. These kinds of conversations are hard to think about. I appreciate that it is simply unacceptable that we have to consider such things. Let's focus on your pain.	*Confirms another conversation, empathizes, and returns as promised to symptoms.*

When patients talk about talking about it, it's important to acknowledge that effort, small though it may seem: Tremendous effort is needed to confront existential fears. For the same reason, we don't think of ourselves as bad clinicians when a patient cannot plan for end of life. Our job is invite but not force participation.

Figure 4.3 shows how to integrate these communication skills into clinical practice. Hesitant patients may need several approaches. One memorable

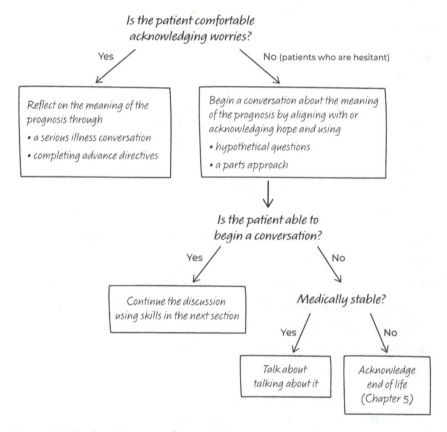

Figure 4.3 The clinical practice of beginning a conversation to deepen prognostic awareness

example was Mike. In his 50s with metastatic lung cancer, Mike couldn't believe that he would die from his cancer even though his oncologist had explained his prognosis several times. His palliative care clinician had asked about the "what ifs" and a worried part, but Mike always answered that he was going to beat the odds. He also had no interest in talking about talking about it: "I've got to keep my focus on the positive." Searching for a cure, he traveled to top medical centers around the country. After one trip, he came to the palliative care clinic complaining of fatigue aggravated by the travel. His clinician asked again whether a part of him worried—worried about traveling so much or missing time with family. The question deepened Mike's prognostic awareness.

"You really think I am going to die from this?"
"Yes," said his clinician.

"Then why am I wasting my time traveling all around the country when I should be with my family?"

Mike's deeper understanding of his prognosis changed his priorities. He received the rest of his cancer treatment locally and spent his remaining time at home with family.

THROUGHOUT THE CONVERSATION

Once the conversation has been started, perhaps with the hypothetical or parts approaches discussed earlier, we continue the conversation by exploring the conversation themes discussed earlier in this chapter. Such conversations help patients to integrate the meaning of the prognosis. This integration makes the patient's experience of the illness more coherent, with thoughts about the prognosis and associated feelings joined into a narrative. To support this integration, we discuss four approaches: exploring, interpreting, allowing feelings to flow, and checking in.

Exploring

Exploring invites the patient to make the unsaid explicit, generating substance for integration. We invite the patient to do most of the talking and sustain the conversation by expressing interest in learning what the patient says.

Exploring is commonly done using "Tell me more." This request can be used to explore thoughts or feelings. With feelings: "You said it broke your heart to be honest with your family. Can you tell me more about that experience?" With thoughts: "Can you tell me more about how you prepared your family?" A variation is exploring extremes: "What is the most difficult part of this?" "Who are you most worried about?" "What frightens you the most?" Finally, we can broaden the exploration using "what else" questions: "What else is on your mind?" or "What else are you worried about?"

Exploring can also be done by reflecting back a portion of what the patient has just said. In choosing that portion, we help guide the conversation. If the patient says, "I had really wanted to go to the beach, and now

I just feel so disappointed," we can highlight and repeat back: "You wanted to go to the beach." This reflection might lead to brainstorming ways to get there or alternative trips. Or we can highlight the feelings: "You feel disappointed." This reflection might lead to an exploration of the other disappointments of a serious illness.

Interpreting

After exploring and surfacing experiences, we interpret: We clarify and synthesize stated or unstated meanings. Interpreting helps patients construct a narrative. Interpreting extends beyond naming unsaid feelings to include clarifying and synthesizing experiences and uncompleted thoughts.

Many clinicians are familiar with naming, making an educated guess about what the patient is feeling and checking by asking or wondering. For example, if a patient says, "I don't want to think about things right now. It's too much," we can name an unsaid feeling: "I wonder if these things are frightening to talk about." We could also interpret an uncompleted thought: "I can see there is a lot on your mind. I wonder if you are trying to figure out how to talk about all of this."

Often, as just illustrated, the clinician interprets a small segment of the conversation. Other times we will listen and explore for a while before interpreting. With one patient, the clinician spoke with the patient for half an hour, learning about the patient's plans for treating new brain metastases, getting updated on the patient's daughter's wedding plans, and hearing about how things were at work. At the end of this conversation, the clinician interpreted the patient's experience: "You are modeling for your children how to face challenging circumstances. They are watching how you manage this and will learn from you. Your courage and grace in this will be part of your legacy to them."

As in any therapeutic relationship, we worry about interpreting incorrectly and breaking rapport. Fortunately, there are ways to repair the relationship, and the benefits in developing connection with the patient are significant. Interpreting, correctly or incorrectly, shows our interest in our patient and that we do not fear unspoken thoughts or feelings. When we interpret correctly, we strengthen the relationship by demonstrating our understanding of the patient's perspective. When we interpret incorrectly, most patients simply correct us: "I am not frightened. It is just too sad to think about." Patients may also correct us nonverbally. Either way, we repair the relationship: "I guessed that you were frightened but I wonder if I got it wrong. Can you tell me more about what you were feeling?" Patients appreciate it when we try again, and the repaired relationship can feel even more connected and attuned than if we had simply interpreted correctly. As one colleague likes to say, "It's about connection, not perfection."

As we remind our trainees and ourselves: Just as a surgeon must tolerate removing an occasional healthy appendix to avoid missing any infected ones, so must the palliative care clinician tolerate interpreting incorrectly. If we never interpret incorrectly, we are not interpreting enough.

Allowing Feelings to Flow

While exploring and interpreting, we offer the patient breaks for feelings to flow. Silence gives patients time to experience feelings. During these pauses, we signal nonverbally that we are still paying attention, can bear the patient's strong emotions, and can even hear more. We also use brief empathic responses to signal our willingness to share in difficult feelings: "I wish things were different," or "I can't imagine how devastating this must be," or even the simple "This is so hard." When feelings have time to flow, patients grieve the many small and large losses that accompany serious illness and live more easily with it.

Checking In

Because these conversations are difficult, we check in now and then with the patient about continuing: "We have talked about a lot today. Is it okay for us to keep talking, or should we take a break and pick this up next time?" We check in also about the content: "We have been talking a lot about your emotions related to the illness. I just wanted to check in to see if this conversation is okay?"

An implicit check-in comes from being aware of patients' nonverbal signs of engagement (nodding, leaning toward us, making notes, or calling family members to join) or disengagement (long pauses, short answers).

A patient-centered way of checking in is through the box metaphor. We introduce it near the beginning of the conversation: "Thinking or talking about the future is like opening a box. You can decide when to open the box, how long to hold it open, and when to close it." When patients feel overwhelmed, they can use it to stop the conversation: "I think we need to close the box now." Or we can use it to check in: "I can see this is getting intense. We could close the box or keep talking. What do you think?" The patient or clinician can also use it to introduce a follow-up conversation: "Could we open that box again today?" The image of the box holding the difficult thoughts and emotions implies that they are not gone, simply safely contained for later exploration. Thus, closing the box does not mean never talking about the future, only that it is time to stop on that day.

One young patient, Chris, became extremely overwhelmed whenever his oncologist made mention of the seriousness of the cancer. When the oncologist tried to review scans or even discuss treatment options, Chris would sob on the exam table, unable to engage in any conversation about what to do. He needed help to contain his emotion so that he could take part in his own medical care. To help Chris control the conversation's intensity, his palliative care clinician introduced the box metaphor so that Chris could stop the conversation when he felt at all overwhelmed. As a way of talking about talking about it, the patient and clinician also considered when to open the box and with whom. In addition, the clinician treated the patient for depression and encouraged him to bring his sister to visits for extra support. Over several months, by opening the box for just a few minutes at a time, Chris learned enough distress tolerance to take part in his medical care.

Closing the Conversation

Sometimes, a conversation becomes overwhelming, and we need to stop it quickly. Our goal is not for this to happen, but sometimes it does. It can happen when we focus on emotions too much or, paradoxically, when patients *think* too much about the illness experience. For example, some patients want to plan their funeral or think about what will happen in the dying process. But if we talk too long or too in depth, this planning or thinking creates hard-to-manage feelings. Even when patients initiate the conversation, they may misjudge their capacity.

Or we can misjudge. One of us was in the room with an oncologist when a patient was told that her disease was incurable. After the oncologist left, the patient was crying, and the clinician reflected, "I can see how terribly sad and overwhelming it is that we can't take this cancer away." To which the patient replied, "Get out. I don't want to talk to you." Naming the unsaid feelings increased the conversation's emotional intensity too far. In retrospect, the clinician reflected that exploring might have been gentler: "I can see this is so upsetting. What is the most upsetting part right now?" When we make a mistake in a difficult situation, sometimes the best thing that we can do is to leave and try again another day.

Here we offer three particularly frequent and useful conversation closers: changing the topic, naming the patient's topic change, and wrapping up.

Changing the Topic

If the conversation is becoming too overwhelming, we privately decide to change to a less charged topic. We first acknowledge the patient's emotion or experience and then direct the conversation, often to symptom management: "It can be overwhelming to think about the future. Let's switch topics and focus on your pain." Other useful focuses include the following:

- The very near future: "This is a lot to think about. What are your plans for today? What are you going to do when you leave here and get home?"
- Achievable hopes and goals: "I can see this is difficult to think about. Tell me about some of the things that you are looking forward to in the next few weeks."
- A recent good event: "You have done a lot of hard thinking today. I am so glad that you enjoyed the beach with your family this past weekend. Good times are so important."

Name the Patient's Topic Change

Sometimes patients change the topic. Then we name the patient's topic change: "Yes, let's change the topic and focus on your pain." Naming the change shows empathy and models how you and the patient can negotiate difficult conversations. It also shows patients that the clinician is monitoring and gently guiding the conversation, which can help them feel contained and secure.

Wrapping Up

Topic changes help us and the patient stop the conversation quickly but are hopefully not needed. Most of the time, we wrap up the conversation once patients give subtle cues that they have had enough discussion for the day (or we need to stop for time management reasons). We signal an ending by praising the patient for the effort: "It is not easy to think about what lies ahead with this illness. You have shown a lot of strength." We then summarize the conversation: "We have talked about some important things, especially how to prepare your family." Our summary is another opportunity for us to interpret the patient's experience. Finally, we mention future work: "Next time, perhaps we should talk about medical decisions that you might face as you get sicker?" Statements of partnership and non-abandonment can also help to close the conversation: "I am not going anywhere. We will keep talking and figure this out."

Tips for Helping Patients Deepen Prognostic Awareness

WHY

Patients cope better and are more prepared for medical and personal decision-making when they reflect on the meaning of the prognosis.

WHEN

Ideally, begin these conversations when patients have met the first three challenges and are still clinically stable.

WHAT

Invite a conversation about the meaning of the prognosis.

For patients comfortable acknowledging worries: Begin a serious illness conversation about hopes, worries, and what's most important and then complete advance directives.

For patients hesitant to talk about worries: Begin the conversation by aligning with or acknowledging hope and explore worries with

- hypothetical questions: "Have you thought about the '*what ifs*' with this cancer?"
- a parts approach: "Is there *a part of you* that worries about what lies ahead?"
- talking about talking about it: who, where, when, advantages, and disadvantages of a conversation about the future (Table 4.2).

Continue the conversation by

- exploring: "Tell me more" or "What is the hardest part?" or "What else?"
- interpreting the patient's experience: "It sounds like this illness has made you parent in a different way that is even better. Is that right?"
- allowing feelings to flow: "I wish things were different."
- checking in: "Should we keep talking or take a break?"

Close the conversation by

- changing topics: Empathize and then focus on symptoms, the near future, hopes and goals, or good things that have happened: "It's hard to think about the future. Let's focus on your symptoms."
- naming the patient's topic change: "I hear you would like to switch focus. We can talk about this another time. Let's get you to infusion."
- wrapping up: praise the patient's effort, summarize, mention future work, and align: "You have shown a lot of strength today in thinking through how to prepare your family. Next time we can talk about how to tell your wishes to your medical team. We will figure this out together."

COLLABORATING WITH COLLEAGUES

The techniques described in this chapter allow palliative care clinicians to help patients deepen their awareness of their prognosis. This growing awareness can be subtle and intermittent, and not always visible to the whole treatment team.

For example, although Sonya initially wouldn't talk about the future, wanting to focus only on the positive, her prognostic awareness deepened as she adapted to her cancer. Her clinician invited her to talk about talking it and used a parts approach. Gradually, Sonya began to mention her longing for her deceased son and how she would see him again soon. Her clinician was reassured that Sonya was acknowledging worries and could have more detailed prognostic conversations with her medical team.

However, when Sonya met with her oncologist, she still focused solely on treatment, speaking only about "getting through this." This positive focus worried the oncologist, who interpreted it as Sonya's unreadiness for conversations about the prognosis and disease trajectory. Yet, the palliative care clinician wasn't as worried. Prognostic awareness changes from context to context and moment to moment. A patient can show good prognostic awareness with palliative care yet not with other members of the medical team. Given this fluidity, different members of the clinical team often disagree on what the patient understands.

In this context, the palliative care clinician has two important roles. The first is to help the patient gradually take in the prognostic information in a manner that is not overwhelming (as described in this chapter). The second is to help the oncologist and the entire medical team understand the patient's prognostic awareness and how it will likely change over time. Thus, when oncology colleagues are frustrated that their patients don't understand the prognosis, despite many detailed conversations and palliative care visits, we remind our colleagues that they have conveyed the prognostic information, and well; it's just that the patient is still swinging on the pendulum.

Even so, Sonya's oncologist had reason to be concerned. Her cancer had progressed quickly on first-line treatment, and she was losing weight on second-line treatment. She was scheduled to have scans within 3 weeks, and the oncologist anticipated that the scans would show cancer progression despite treatment. If so, he anticipated a conversation about hospice in the upcoming weeks or months and wanted to prepare Sonya. The clinicians planned a joint visit.

Joint visits are particularly helpful when clinicians worry that a patient has low prognostic awareness or when clinicians have different perspectives on the patient's prognostic awareness (as in Sonya's case). Sonya's joint visit showed the palliative care clinician how difficult the oncologist's situation was. Although Sonya could be vulnerable in palliative care visits, she blocked the oncologist's attempts to talk about the future during the joint visit. Asking many questions about medications and side effects of chemotherapy, she left little opportunity for either clinician to talk about the future.

After the visit, the clinicians debriefed about how Sonya's focus on treatment precluded a deeper discussion. It was probably scary for Sonya to talk about getting sicker with the clinician who held the keys to treatment. The clinicians agreed that, because Sonya could be vulnerable in palliative care visits, those visits would be the place to explore her fears.

When debriefing after a joint visit we tread lightly. We acknowledge how difficult the end-of-life transition is and affirm the oncologist's skill because we know our colleagues can feel self-conscious with us in the room watching. During debriefs, our colleagues sometimes ask for feedback about their communication approach. We always start with a successful moment: "I just want to acknowledge how caring you were in there. I think the patient felt your deep investment, and it was comforting." We also give specific examples: "When you said, 'I can see this is overwhelming,' that was very skilled. You noticed how she was feeling. You stopped what you were saying, and then you named her emotion. I think that allowed her to reflect on the information." By identifying moments of effective communication, we can give language to what might have been an intuitive response and strengthen a skill.

Reflecting on successful moments builds a foundation to reflect gently on the challenges. We might ask the oncologist, "What was the toughest part for you?" We often suggest concrete language that might have helped: "Sometimes when patients are overwhelmed, I need to use several empathic statements to offer comfort. I have found it helpful to say, 'I wish I had better news.'" Finally, to foster our own learning, we ask the oncologist for what *we* might have done differently.

MEETING THE CHALLENGE OF DEEPENING PROGNOSTIC AWARENESS

In this chapter, we discussed how to have difficult conversations with patients about the meaning of the prognosis. Some patients are readier for these goals and values conversations, which might then be done by the oncologist or primary care clinician. Other patients need specialist palliative care support to build distress tolerance. These conversations are best held when patients are still feeling well, before the illness progresses and forces more urgent medical decisions.

Patients have met this challenge of deepening prognostic awareness when they can talk about and plan for the possibility of dying. Each patient will have unique preferences about how much to know, how much to talk about it, and how detailed the planning should be. Over time, as patients build distress tolerance, their information preferences and capacity for these conversations evolve.

Once patients have met this challenge, we return to a focus on living well (Chapter 3). The positive focus of living well balances the strong emotions of these prognostic awareness conversations. We often move back and forth between living well and deepening prognostic awareness within one visit, depending on the patient's distress tolerance and on the clinical situation. If the illness is progressing and the patient seems unprepared for getting sicker, we focus more on this challenge. But when the illness has progressed such that medical decisions need to be made imminently, we move to the fifth challenge: acknowledging end of life.

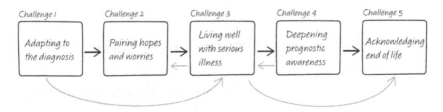

COMMUNICATION SKILLS SUMMARY

CHAPTER 1: ADAPTING TO THE DIAGNOSIS

Assess prognostic awareness: What is your understanding of your illness? Looking to the future, what are your hopes? What are your worries?

Support coping: Normalize, align, contain.

Be an interpreter: Interpret the patient for the oncologist and the oncologist for the patient.

CHAPTER 2: PAIRING HOPES AND WORRIES

For patients who focus solely on hope: Align with hope and touch upon the illness by

- empathizing
- understanding the illness's impact on others
- suggesting a worried part
- mentioning the "what ifs"
- linking to worries with "even though"

For patients who acknowledge hopes and worries: Pair the patient's hopes and worries, and normalize these mixed feelings.

CHAPTER 3: LIVING WELL WITH SERIOUS ILLNESS

Promote healthy coping by

- exploring what it means to live well with the illness
- asking how patients have coped and are coping
- introducing new skills to broaden the patient's repertoire (behavioral, cognitive, emotional, existential)

CHAPTER 4: DEEPENING PROGNOSTIC AWARENESS

For patients who can pair hopes and worries: Invite a serious illness conversation about hopes, worries, and what's important, and then complete advance directives.

For patients hesitant to talk about worries:

- Begin the conversation by aligning with or acknowledging hope and explore worries with hypothetical questions, a parts approach, or talking about talking about it.
- Continue the conversation by exploring, interpreting the patient's experience, allowing feelings to flow, and checking in.
- Close the conversation by changing topics, naming the patient's topic change, and wrapping up.

Further Reading

Back, A. L., Arnold, R. M., Baile, W. F., Fryer-Edwards, K. A., Alexander, S. C., Barley, G. E., Gooley, T. A., & Tulsky, J. A. (2007). Efficacy of communication skills training for giving bad news and discussing transitions to palliative care. *Archives of Internal Medicine, 167*(5), 453–460.

Bernacki, R., Block, S., & American College of Physicians High Value Care Task Force. (2014). Communication about serious illness care goals: A review and synthesis of best practices. *JAMA Internal Medicine, 174*(12), 1994–2003.

Bernacki, R., Hutchings, M., Vick, J., Smith, G., Paladino, J., Lipsitz, S., Gawande, A. A., & Block, S. D. (2015). Development of the serious illness care program: A randomised controlled trial of a palliative care communication intervention. *BMJ Open, 5*(10), e009032.

Butow, P. N., Brown, R. F., Cogar, S., Tattersall, M. H., & Dunn, S. M. (2002). Oncologists' reactions to cancer patients' verbal cues. *Psycho-Oncology, 11*(1), 47–58.

Jackson, V. A., Jacobsen, J., Greer, J. A., Pirl, W. F., Temel, J. S., & Back, A. L. (2013). The cultivation of prognostic awareness through the provision of early palliative care in the ambulatory setting: A communication guide. *Journal of Palliative Medicine, 16*(8), 894–900.

Jacobsen, J., Blinderman, C., Alexander Cole, C., & Jackson, V. (2018). "I'd recommend . . .": How to incorporate your recommendation into shared decision making for patients with serious illness. *Journal of Pain and Symptom Management, 55*(4), 1224–1230.

Jacobsen, J., Brenner, K., Greer, J. A., Jacobo, M., Rosenberg, L., Nipp, R. D., & Jackson, V. A. (2018). When a patient is reluctant to talk about it: A dual framework to focus on living well and tolerate the possibility of dying. *Journal of Palliative Medicine, 21*(3), 322–327.

Jacobsen, J., Thomas, J. D., & Jackson, V. A. (2013). Misunderstandings about prognosis: An approach for palliative care consultants when the patient does not seem to understand what was said. *Journal of Palliative Medicine, 16*(1), 91–95.

Jacobsen, J., Tran, K. M., Jackson, V. A., & Rubin, E. B. (2020). Case 19-2020: A 74-year-old man with acute respiratory failure and unclear goals of care. *New England Journal of Medicine, 382*, 2450–2457.

Pollak, K. I., Childers, J. W., & Arnold, R. M. (2011). Applying motivational interviewing techniques to palliative care communication. *Journal of Palliative Medicine, 14*(5), 587–592.

Prendergast, T. J. (2001). Advance care planning: Pitfalls, progress, promise. *Critical Care Medicine, 29*(2, Suppl.), N34–N39.

Rietjens, J. A. C., Sudore, R. L., Connolly, M., van Delden, J. J., Drickamer, M. A., Droger, M., van der Heide, A., Heyland, D. K., Houttekier, D., Janssen, D. J. A., Orsi, L., Payne, S., Seymour, J., Jox, R. J., Korfage, I. J.; European Association for Palliative Care. (2017). Definition and recommendations for advance care planning: An international consensus supported by the European Association for Palliative Care. *Lancet Oncology, 18*(9), e543–e551.

Suchman, A. L., Markakis, K., Beckman, H. B., & Frankel, R. (1997). A model of empathic communication in the medical interview. *Journal of the American Medical Association, 277*(8), 678–682.

Sudore, R. L., Lum, H. D., You, J. J., Hanson, L. C., Meier, D. E., Pantilat, S. Z., Matlock, D. D., Rietjens, J. A. C., Korfage, I. J., Ritchie, C. S., Kutner, J. S., Teno, J. M., Thomas, J., McMahan, R. D., & Heyland, D. K. (2017). Defining advance care planning for adults: A consensus definition from a multidisciplinary Delphi panel. *Journal of Pain and Symptom Management, 53*(5), 821–832.

Tolle, S. W., & Teno, J. M. (2018, July 19). Counting POLST form completion can hinder quality. *Health Affairs Blog.* doi:10.1377/hblog20180709.244065

Yadav, K. N., Gabler, N. B., Cooney, E., Kent, S., Kim, J., Herbst, N., Mante, A., Halpern, S. D., & Courtright, K. R. (2017). Approximately one in three US adults completes any type of advance directive for end-of-life care. *Health Affairs, 36*(7), 1244–1251.

Acknowledging End of Life

Carlos, the patient with colon cancer introduced in Chapter 3, had been de-
pendent on total parenteral nutrition for almost a year. Now, he was tired,
depressed, and getting weaker. He lived at home, where he could spend time
with his teenage children.

Carlos had healthy prognostic awareness. He spoke of the incurability of
his cancer and of his worries for his wife and children. He set realistic goals,
such as attending his son's graduation. Despite his depression, he fostered
good family times such as game nights.

Although Carlos seemed prepared for end of life, he wanted to try new
treatments even as his functional status declined significantly. Because he
had been sick for so long, he had adapted to his low performance status and
could not recognize that he was close to end of life.

THE CHALLENGE OF ACKNOWLEDGING END OF LIFE

A palliative care clinician working for a long time with a patient like Carlos
faces a hard task. Carlos believes strongly that more treatment is the only
option, which puts pressure on his oncologist to provide treatments that
may hold little benefit. The palliative care clinician wants to help Carlos
more clearly understand his medical situation so that he can make
decisions that align with his values.

As their illness progresses, patients like Carlos face the fifth challenge: acknowledging end of life. This acknowledgment may be an overt discussion about dying. It may also be indirect, using allusions and euphemisms. Clinicians need not say the "D-word" in order to help patients meet the fifth challenge. Clinicians and patients just need to share an implicit understanding.

In order to acknowledge end of life, patients must develop the worried part of themselves (Figure 5.1). They then see their prognosis more clearly and can use this understanding to make medical and personal decisions about how to live at the very end of life.

Even when patients have built coping skills and deepened their prognostic awareness, this acknowledgment of end of life does not always happen spontaneously. It usually requires another factor: attuned communication from the medical team. In this chapter, we discuss communication skills to help patients acknowledge end of life. We also explore how

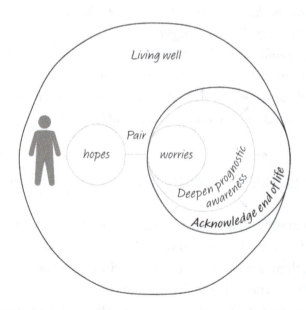

Figure 5.1 Adding challenge 5: acknowledging end of life. As patients acknowledge end of life, their prognostic awareness deepens, and the worries circle again expands.

a patient nearing end of life can create tensions within the medical team and how these tensions can be eased.

Maintaining Attunement as Patients Get Sicker

Maintaining attunement with patients as they approach the end of life can be difficult. They still cope in the healthy pattern of swinging between hopes and worries and therefore have conflicting emotional and informational needs: wanting honest information to prepare for the future while wanting to preserve hope. This fluctuation becomes more difficult for us as patients get sicker. When our patient was medically stable, we could follow the patient's lead. We aligned with hopes and talked about worries only when the patient could accept more difficult conversations. However, when our patient gets sicker, the illness sets its own agenda. Attuned to the whole patient, including physical state, we must hold these conversations to guide medical decision-making, even if the patient is not ready. In this situation, many clinicians worry about compromising clinical attunement. But the strong relationship we have built with the patient through facing the preceding challenges helps us stay connected even as we discuss unwelcome information.

Palliative Care Discussions at the End of Life

As patients become sicker, a significant part of our role is guiding them and their families through end-of-life decision-making. To understand this process, members of our team, led by Dr. Lara Traeger, analyzed audio-recorded study visits to characterize palliative care communication patterns. This research revealed three important communication themes in how clinicians maintain attunement as patients approach end of life.

Theme 1: As clinicians see that the patient is not tolerating treatment, they encourage the patient and family to consider the quality-of-life implications of treatment. The following dialog illustrates this (light) encouragement.

Bringing up quality-of-life values

CLINICIAN: I think that's the tradeoff. Does the treatment improve my quality of life? It will give me a little bit more time, but what kind of time is it? And when is it maybe not worth it? And what else is important?

PATIENT: [Oncologist] said that we'll give the chemotherapy a try. I say fine.

CLINICIAN: I think that's fine, fingers crossed. I hope this goes easier for you.

When the patient resists quality-of-life considerations, as illustrated here, clinicians often align with the decision ("I think that's fine") and leave open the possibility that the course might shift at some point ("fingers crossed"). Aligning with the decision maintains an emotional connection with the patient. Leaving open the possibility for change helps the clinician gently guide the patient toward anticipated decision-making. As another clinician phrased it, "I think that is a perfectly reasonable thing to do, and I think it's important that, if there comes a time when it feels like it's too much, we can have a discussion about that."

Theme 2: As patients become sicker, conversations become more frank and focus on end-of-life decisions. For example, one palliative care clinician was frank not only about the patient's condition but also about his own reaction to the patient's decline: "When I called you a few weeks ago, your health had changed so quickly. I was shocked. I think it even took me a little bit of time to catch how quickly it changed, so I can imagine what it must be like for your family." Clinicians also draw on information from prior discussions to make more explicit recommendations: "You have been saying for months the most important thing to you is your family, and being around your kids, and probably being home. I think this is the time to get you home."

Theme 3: Visits include candid, reflective, and intimate exchanges between patients and families and their clinicians. As time grows shorter, patients, families, and clinicians share experiences, anecdotes, dark humor, or reflections, indicating a deeper and more trusting relationship.

Connecting

PATIENT: My 16-year-old grandchild sat with me and rubbed my back. I said to him, "Don't do that." He said, "Why?" I said, "Because you'll make me cry." And he rubbed my back. I said to him, "Thank you very much for taking care of me Saturday night." And he said, "It's no problem, Nana, you've been doing it for me all my life."

CLINICIAN: Good kid, huh?

PATIENT: Yeah, real good kid.

Knowing the patient helps clinicians make candid prognostic disclosures and recommendations that sometimes differ from the patient's previous preferences: "We talked a long time ago about you being home for the end, but now I wonder if being at the hospital or at the hospice might give your family a little bit more support."

HOW TO HELP PATIENTS
ACKNOWLEDGE END OF LIFE

It's hard to acknowledge that the cancer will take your life one day. It's harder to acknowledge that this day is near. Furthermore, patients have varying levels of hesitancy about these conversations, even when they have been preparing with us for a long time. When these conversations are triggered by a sudden clinical decline, they can be even more difficult because patients may be feeling poorly or afraid. The following sections discuss skills for holding an attuned conversation about end of life.

Asking Asking Asking Before Telling

Our conversation will be guided by what the patient already knows, is ready to hear, and finds helpful. These aspects are built into an approach that we call Ask-Ask-Ask-Tell-Ask. It extends the Ask-Tell-Ask strategy for discussing bad news: asking the patient to describe his or her current understanding of the issue (Ask), discussing the information accordingly (Tell), and asking the patient to repeat what was heard (Ask). With Ask-Ask-Ask-Tell-Ask, the first Ask step expands to a series of questions (Ask-Ask-Ask). It reminds us to ask many questions to understand what the patient knows and wants to know before acknowledging end of life (Tell).

The exact order or combination of questions is not essential, and not all questions need to be asked. The basic groupings (Box 5.1) are Ask (for illness understanding), Ask (for information preferences), and Ask (for permission).

Hearing many questions, the patient might think we are avoiding the tough conversation. Thus, we often preface our questions with an

Box 5.1 ASK-ASK-ASK QUESTIONS

Illness understanding

"What is your sense of the future?"

"What have you and the oncologist discussed about the big picture?"

"What is your body telling you about what is happening?"

Information preferences

"Some people want a lot of details about what lies ahead; others prefer having the big picture. What kind of information is most helpful to you?"

"Some people want to know how much time they may have; others are more interested in what that time might be like. What type of prognostic information is most helpful for you?"

"What are the benefits of having more prognostic information?"

"Are there downsides to having more prognostic information?"

Permission

"Would it be okay if I shared my sense of what lies ahead?"

"Would it be helpful if I talk about what happens to most people in the dying process?"

explanation of their need: "I am worried that we need to talk about what lies ahead, yet I do not know how much information would be most helpful. Would it be okay if I asked some questions so that I can be sure to give you the right information?"

The following example illustrates this approach with Carlos. Although the clinician knows Carlos well, she still uses the Ask-Ask-Ask approach to learn more about what he understands and wants to know.

Getting ready to talk with Carlos about the prognosis

DIALOG	OUR PRESPECTIVE
CARLOS: Well, I made it—had to use one of these today (points to the wheelchair). I just can't seem to shake this fatigue.	
CLINICIAN: It sounds like your body is struggling.	
CARLOS: I just feel so tired. Is there a pill that can help with this? I know I need to be strong for treatment. I can't keep going like this.	
CLINICIAN: Carlos, I know that you want to feel better and have more treatment. I am also very worried about how you are doing. Would it be okay to talk more?	*Pairs hope and worry and makes the first ask for permission.*
CARLOS: Sure, I guess.	
CLINICIAN: Carlos, what is your sense of the future?	*Second ask, for illness understanding.*
CARLOS: More chemotherapy, I guess. I know that I am not going to live forever, but a little more time would be nice.	
CLINICIAN: What is your body telling you now?	*Third ask, for illness understanding.*
CARLOS: My body is done. It can't take much more.	
CLINICIAN: I am worried about that too. How much do you want to know about what lies ahead?	*Fourth ask, for information preferences.*

Dialog	Our perspective
CARLOS: I had a bad feeling this conversation was coming. Is it really time to talk about this?	
CLINICIAN: I think we should begin the conversation.	
CARLOS: What do you think? How much time do I have?	*Despite some initial reluctance, Carlos transitions to a conversation about the prognosis.*
CLINICIAN: I hear that you want to know more about how much time remains. Would it be helpful to have specific information or a better sense of the big picture?	*Fifth ask, for more detailed information preferences.*
CARLOS: I think let's start with the big picture.	

In this conversation, the clinician learns that Carlos is hoping for a little more time but realizes that his body cannot withstand more treatment. In our research, we found that patients' perceptions of their health status are a significant predictor of survival. We don't mean that negative thoughts somehow hamper survival. Rather, when patients report that they are seriously ill, they are tapping into an accurate internal sense of their bodily state. Knowing this sense is accurate gives us confidence to start a frank discussion about end of life.

Pairing Hope with Worry

Once we understand what prognostic information would be most helpful, we can discuss the prognosis. The most attuned approach reprises the approach introduced in Chapter 2, pairing hope and worry, allowing for hope among distressing prognostic information.

We usually make this pairing within one sentence: "I hear you are hoping to feel better and have more treatment, and I am worried that your body is getting weaker and that time is short." An important grammatical caveat is to join the hope and the worry with "and" rather than "but." As one of us says when teaching, "If my husband says, 'You look great, but I'm not sure that those shoes go with that dress.' I feel worse than if he says, 'You look great, and I'm not sure that those shoes go with that dress.'" Using "but" negates the hope, and (sorry!) using "and" allows the ideas to coexist. When we are very worried, the "but" sometimes slips out anyway because, in our hearts, we do not feel much hope. We try to avoid this error.

Yet when patients are very sick, how do we find a hope with which the patient can also align? Depending on the situation, we might align with a patient's hope for a miracle or for comfort. Sometimes we simply hope that we are wrong: "I am hoping that I am wrong, and I am worried that time is very short." A variation is to pair a wish with the worry: "I wish for better news, and I worry that time is very short."

Layering the Prognostic Disclosure

When pairing hope and worry, we often use a layered or titrated approach. We make a general prognostic statement and assess how much more to say by how the patient reacts. The layers can include a preparatory warning ("I wish things were different. I have some bad news to share") followed by a general statement ("I worry that time may be shorter than we hoped"). Then we'd check in to see what more the patient wants to know. If it is length of time, we might add, "I worry time may be as short as days to a few weeks." If it is what that time might be like, we might offer, "I worry that this fatigue and weakness is only going to get worse."

With Carlos, this layered approach lets him decide how much to hear. Throughout the discussion, the clinician offers empathic statements and refrains from backtracking.

Using a layered approach to discuss prognostic information with Carlos

DIALOG	OUR PRESPECTIVE
CARLOS: I think, let's start with the big picture.	
CLINICIAN: I wish for better news, and I worry that time may be short.	*Pairs hope and worry to introduce a general prognostic statement.*
CARLOS: That is what I was worried about.	
CLINICIAN: Would it be helpful to talk more specifically about how much time remains?	*Checks in with Carlos by asking how much more he wants to know.*
CARLOS: Yes, I want to know whatever you think. I need to make plans.	
CLINICIAN: I am hoping that I am wrong, and I worry that time may be as short as weeks to a small number of months.	*Clarifies the prognostic estimate.*
CARLOS: Really? I did not think it would be so soon.	
CLINICIAN: I can't imagine how hard this is to hear.	*Avoids backtracking, for example by discussing the uncertainties of a prognosis, and instead responds empathically.*

When using a layered approach, we don't always ask the patient in advance for detailed information preferences. Instead, based on our clinical judgment of the patient's coping, we might privately decide how much more to disclose. For example, if we disclose that time is short and our patient becomes upset and wants to plan for hospice, the patient probably understands enough to make decisions and doesn't need explicit detail about how much time remains. Our long relationship with patients often informs these attuned decisions. For example, if the patient asked for more information or we knew the patient as a detail-oriented person who wanted specifics, we would disclose more.

Layering is particularly needed when a patient's illness is progressing quickly, leaving limited time to adapt to difficult news. We then check in with the patient throughout the disclosure to ensure that the patient is getting enough information without becoming overwhelmed. These check-ins can be observational, watching how the patient is coping with the prognostic information. They can also be questions: "Are you doing okay?" or "Would it be helpful to know more?" Check-ins can also be empathic statements: "I wish I had better news" or "I can't imagine what it must be like to hear this news."

These check-ins give patients time to process emotions and to reassess their information preferences. We sometimes preface this process by saying, "As I discuss what lies ahead, I will check in with you so that I can be sure I am giving you the right amount of information. Some people find the big picture to be enough; others want more specific information. Everyone is different. You don't need to know very specific information in order to plan well."

Throughout the conversation, we support the patient using empathic statements and silence. The patient or family members may understandably become sad or angry. At this critical juncture in our relationship, patients need us to withstand their strong emotions and to hold fast to our understanding of the prognosis. Based on this understanding, patients can then make medical decisions.

Yet, even with years of experience, we can easily feel tempted to soften or retract the prognostic information just discussed. We might explain how uncertain a prognosis can be. Or, when the suggestion of hospice angers a family, we might backtrack and discuss a bridge program. Trainees often backtrack by providing more biomedical information about the disease, treatment, or side effects, which distracts the conversation away from the prognosis. Backtracking is sometimes necessary to preserve a relationship with the patient or family but should ideally be avoided. Fortunately, as we developed stronger empathic communication skills, we needed to backtrack less often.

Empathic communication depends on fluency with empathic statements and on cognitive comfort with strong feelings: a way of thinking about the patient's strong feelings that helps us respond with empathic statements rather than react by backtracking. Thus, we might say to ourselves that the patient's strong feelings are okay: "This patient is angry and sad because the news that I just shared is terrible, not because I said it badly. I can help this patient bear these feelings. I don't need to change what I said." We are applying cognitive restructuring and self-efficacy (discussed in Chapter 3) to ourselves.

Naming the Dilemma

But what if a very sick patient cannot talk about the big picture? This situation happens even with early integrated palliative care. When an illness progresses very rapidly, patients might not have enough time to build distress tolerance. Or, when patients have been stable for a long time, they may not easily understand that the illness has progressed. Some patients have very optimistic family members who inhibit patients from talking about the future. We have also seen young patients struggle to adapt to the prognosis. Finally, patients like Carlos, who have met all four challenges, may simply have trouble taking the difficult last step of acknowledging end of life.

When a patient is not integrating prognostic information and time is short, the clinician and patient can become polarized. On the one side is the patient, focused on treatments, staying positive, and getting through the illness. On the other side is the palliative care or oncology clinician, increasingly worried that treatments are unlikely to provide benefit and could even do harm. Everybody feels stuck.

To ease this stalemate and maintain attunement, we metaphorically place ourselves alongside the patient, looking at the problem of the illness. The problem is neither the patient who cannot accept the prognosis, nor the clinician who has given up hope. The problem is the disease, advancing despite everyone's efforts. With this picture in mind, we then name this dilemma for the patient. First, we describe the patient's perspec on the problem and then we discuss our perspective, including our concern about not talking further about the future.

This approach feels directive, especially when patients don't want to talk, and clinicians may themselves hesitate to have the conversation. This hesitation comes from a recognition that patients are vulnerable because they are sick and because of the inherent power difference in the doctor–patient relationship. Pushing patients can also feel hard when there is prognostic uncertainty and we could be wrong. But this conversation is not about us being right about what lies ahead. Rather, it is about helping patients understand that they are very likely approaching end of life and need a more accurate prognostic understanding to make medical and personal decisions.

To illustrate this approach, we return to Carlos. If Carlos had not been able to acknowledge end of life, here is how we might have named the dilemma. The example begins with Carlos (hypothetically) hesitating to talk about getting sicker.

Naming the dilemma with Carlos

DIALOG	OUR PRESPECTIVE
CLINICIAN: What is your body telling you now?	*Third ask, for illness understanding.*
CARLOS: It's telling me it's not time yet, that I still have more fight.	*Hesitates to talk about the future.*
CLINICIAN: Carlos, I know how hard this is to talk about. And I certainly don't want to upset you. I hear that you want to keep fighting and that you just want a bit more time.	*Describes Carlos's perspective as part of naming the dilemma.*

Dialog	Our perspective
CLINICIAN (CONTINUED): At the same time, I am worried. I can see that you are getting weaker. And I wonder whether it is time to think about your priorities if time were short. I worry that, if we don't talk about this, you might miss out on doing things that are important to you.	*Describes the clinician's perspective, including the downside of not talking more.*
CARLOS: I see. I didn't understand things were that serious.	
CLINICIAN: What would be your most important priorities if time were short?	*Begins a goals and values conversation.*

Naming the dilemma enables an attuned conversation about what is happening. Our goal is not to undermine the oncologist or to force the patient off treatment. Our goal is to share our honest assessment and to invite the patient to reflect on what is happening and consider options.

As an aside, we sometimes recommend that our patients name the dilemma with family or other loved ones. One patient was unsure about how much to discuss her illness with her adult son. Her son had avoided these conversations, and the patient suspected that talking about the seriousness of the illness would overwhelm him. But she also worried that she was not preparing him well. We discussed how she could name the dilemma with her son. The patient could say: "On the one hand, I get the sense that this illness is difficult for you to talk about. I want to respect that. I don't want to give you information that is too much to manage. On the other hand, I would like to support you through this. And I am not sure how to do that if we don't discuss what is happening. What are your thoughts?" Using this approach, the patient broached the topic of her illness with her son. Her son did not want more information at that time, but they agreed to check in after each oncology visit.

Making a Recommendation to Ease Decision-Making

Sometimes patients are getting sicker and understand the prognosis but struggle to make medical decisions. These patients seem paralyzed, even though they had been clear with their clinician about what they would want should they get sicker. For these patients, we make recommendations about medical decisions. Our recommendations ease the stress of decision-making, especially for end-of-life care decisions about hospice or resuscitation.

Guiding patients and families through medical decisions—making recommendations—is inherent to medical care. Oncologists consider the patient's functional status and medical history to recommend a chemotherapy approach. As palliative care clinicians, we consider the patient's pain syndrome and medication history to recommend an opioid regimen. Yet, recommending end-of-life care, such as CPR or hospice, seems more directive or even paternalistic because these decisions are so personal. Clinicians therefore often worry about biasing patients or infringing on their autonomy.

However, their autonomy is supported by our recommendations, and these recommendations, research shows, are welcomed by patients and families. By recommending a plan consistent with the prognosis, we help patients and families understand the prognosis and adapt to it. By contrast, neutral questions ("Do you want a visiting nurse or hospice?" "Do you want CPR?") can leave the impression that all options are equal, when we know that some options offer little benefit and can cause harm.

In shared decision-making, clinicians make medical recommendations based on the medical situation and on the patient's goals, values, and preferences. In these latter aspects, patients and families are the experts, while clinicians are the experts in making a recommendation that translates goals, values, and preferences into a treatment plan. Because not all clinicians have used a shared decision-making process that includes making a specific medical recommendation, we offer as guidance the following three steps: (1) reflecting on the options, (2) understanding the patient's goals and values, and (3) synthesizing a recommendation. As an example, we use the recommendation for hospice given to Carlos.

Step 1: Reflecting on the Options

We first understand the prognosis and the likelihood of benefit for any treatments (Box 5.2). Because this information is often uncertain and we are not experts in chemotherapy outcomes, we often consult with the oncologist. Carlos's oncologist agreed that time was short, on the order of weeks to months. In addition, Carlos had no remaining standard chemotherapy options and, because of his low performance status, couldn't qualify for a clinical trial.

We next imagine how treatments would align with a range of different values, so that we have synthesized the medical information in our minds before we talk with the patient. We prepare for two common situations.

Box 5.2 **Consider the Prognosis and Treatment Options**

Understand the prognosis and treatment options
  "How much time remains?"
  "How will the patient's function change?"
  "What would I share if the patient asks?"
  "What treatments could safely be offered that have a reasonable likelihood of benefit?"
  "What is the burden of these treatments?"

**Consider how available options might align with a range
of goals and values**
  "What options maximize quality of life? Length of life?"
  "What options minimize symptom burden?"
  "What options would I recommend to my own family?"
  "On what values are my recommendation based?"

First, many patients value living as well as possible for as long as possible. We plan for how to honor this value. For Carlos, the palliative care clinician confirmed with the oncologist that the best way to maintain Carlos's quality of life for as long as possible would be to stop chemotherapy. (In our research, patients who received early integrated palliative care stopped cytotoxic chemotherapy earlier in the disease trajectory and had more time from their last chemotherapy until their death. Despite these patients stopping chemotherapy earlier, they did not experience worse survival outcomes compared to those receiving usual oncology care.)

Second, many patients and families will ask, "If this were your father, what would you do?" or "If you were in my position, what would you do?" We think through what we would say to this question. It is ethical for clinicians to share their opinion and good practice to explain what values inform the opinion: "I know that my father values being at home, even if it means that he might live for a shorter time. So, if this were my father, I would recommend home hospice."

If Carlos had asked us, "What would you do?" he might have heard, "From my work in palliative care, I have learned that it is important to have a period of letting go. This time helps families to grieve together and adapt, which I think is important. So, if it were me, I would choose hospice because it is a signal that it is time to come together for the last phase. Hospice also gives families support."

STEP 2: UNDERSTANDING THE PATIENT'S GOALS AND VALUES

The second step in making a recommendation is understanding patients' actual goals and values so that we can help them figure out which ones they can realistically maintain. When the clinician asked Carlos what was most important, Carlos said that his priority was his family. The clinician then probed this value with two simple questions (Figure 5.2).

- "Tell me more" encouraged Carlos to elaborate, which deepened the clinician's understanding of the specific value.
- "And what else?" encouraged Carlos to articulate a range of values, and asking it repeatedly increased the range. (Eliciting this range helps particularly when a patient's first priority is not possible.)

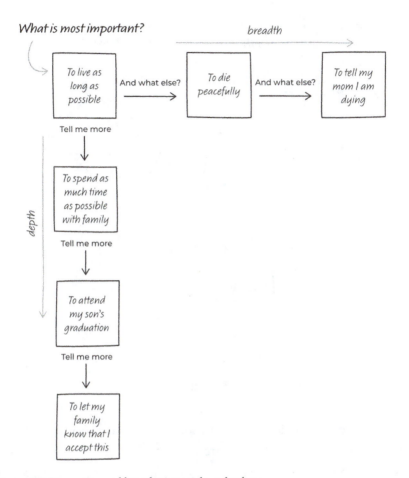

Figure 5.2 Deepening and broadening goals and values

STEP 3: SYNTHESIZING A RECOMMENDATION

Finally, integrating our understanding of the medical options with what is important to our patient, we synthesize a recommendation (Figure 5.3). This synthesis accords with our ethical responsibility to provide guidance and not simply to ask patients what they want.

Before offering any recommendation, it's useful to ask permission: "Would it be helpful if I offered a recommendation?" However, if a patient seems stuck or overwhelmed by the medical options, we skip this step and offer a recommendation based on what we already know about the patient: "I know how important it is for you to support your family through this illness, so, at this point, I recommend . . ."

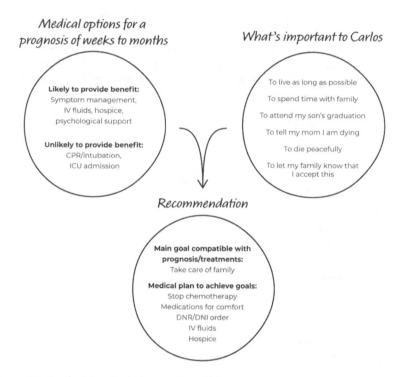

Figure 5.3 Synthesizing Carlos's recommendation

With Carlos, the clinician recommended a plan of care based on Carlos's most important value of taking care of his family. This plan focused on making the most of the time remaining and included medications for his comfort at home, which honored his goal of dying peacefully. It also included supporting Carlos in his goal of trying to attend his son's graduation, including intravenous fluids, if needed. Since resuscitation or chemotherapy was unlikely to give Carlos more time with his family and chemotherapy might even cause harm, the clinician recommended stopping chemotherapy, completing a form to limit resuscitation, and enrolling in hospice.

The clinician's recommendations to Carlos and his family were grounded in the medical literature, which shows many benefits of hospice and bereavement support for caregivers of patients with cancer. These benefits include improved family function, better bereavement adjustment, improved satisfaction, decreased depression, and fewer unmet needs. In a matched cohort study, surviving spouses of patients who died on hospice even lived longer. Patients and families are likely to experience these benefits when they have been enrolled with hospice for enough time. Although the optimal timing for hospice enrollment is unclear, depression symptoms in surviving spouses have been reduced after enrollment for only 3 days.

Even when patients don't accept our recommendations, they continue to meet with us, to seek our opinion, and to trust us because we have established a partnership. They know that we will support them regardless of what medical decisions they make. For example, when we recommend hospice, our patients often say that they are not ready. But our partnership continues, with us as a stabilizing presence providing emotional support and medical expertise through difficult decisions.

Tips for Helping Patients Acknowledge End of Life

WHY

When we talk honestly with sick patients about their illness and prognosis, we give them the information that they need to make medical and personal end-of-life decisions.

WHEN

We hold these conversations when patients are approaching end of life and are at a decision point in their medical care. (We also use the skills for discussing prognosis throughout the illness, when patients ask for prognostic information.)

WHAT

While talking about the future honestly and providing guidance about treatment decisions, we maintain attunement by asking lots of questions and checking in.

Help the patient first acknowledge end of life by

- using Ask-Ask-Ask (before Telling): Ask for illness understanding, for information preferences, and for permission.

- pairing hope with worry using "and": "I am hoping that I am wrong, and I am worried that time may be short."
- layering the prognostic disclosure: "I am worried that time may be short. [pause] It may be as short as a few weeks, perhaps only 2 or 3 weeks."
- naming the dilemma: "On the one hand, I can hear that this is hard to talk about and that you would rather have this conversation another time. On the other hand, I am worried about what is happening with the cancer and that your body is getting very sick. I am worried that your medical team will not know how to take care of you. Can we think together about how we might talk about what lies ahead?"

Then recommend treatment and disposition by (1) reflecting on the options, (2) understanding the patient's values and goals, (3) and synthesizing a recommendation.

COLLABORATING WITH COLLEAGUES

In this chapter, we have focused on how to maintain attunement with patients and families even as the illness forces difficult conversations and decisions. But these conversations are not the only difficult ones. As we guide patients' medical decisions, despite managing role overlap and understanding the clinical goals, we sometimes find ourselves in conflict with the oncologist.

In one common scenario, we disagree with the oncologist about the direction of treatment. For example, the patient receives a new cancer-directed therapy despite a low performance status. When patients are so sick that they are unlikely to benefit from treatment, we worry about the toxicity of another line of therapy. Initiating a new treatment may also give an overly optimistic message about the prognosis, a false hope preventing patients and families from preparing for end-of-life decisions and for the transition to hospice. Making this situation a dilemma, we also worry that an honest discussion with the oncologist would compromise our collegial relationship.

In another common scenario, we think that the oncologist has not adequately communicated the prognosis to the patient so the patient cannot properly decide whether or not to continue treatment. Even knowing the pendulum of prognostic awareness and that patients do not always hear what the oncology team says, we wonder how on earth the patient can have such low prognostic awareness. When the patient then has unrealistic expectations for treatment, developing a unified care plan can be difficult. We feel stuck.

One patient, Helen, illustrates a typical conflict situation. Helen was in her mid-60s with metastatic non-small-cell lung cancer. She had progressed through platinum-based chemotherapy and had developed peritoneal metastases (a rare complication of lung cancer) that caused severe pain. Her pain was difficult to control despite a month-long hospital admission. Feeling relief only when sedated, she slept most of the time and was intermittently delirious. She couldn't interact with her family and experienced ongoing distress from her symptoms. Helen was dying.

When Helen's oncologist wanted to offer a new treatment (immunotherapy), we got worried that additional treatment could worsen her suffering and delay her transition to hospice. It was time for an honest conversation with the oncologist.

Preparing for an Honest Conversation

Before such a conversation, we check in with the rest of the palliative care team or another trusted oncology colleague in order to let our own feelings flow and to confirm our medical assessment. We are then less likely in the conversation itself to be reactive or defensive, and we have a better understanding of the treatment options. Cancer care evolves rapidly and staying current with new treatments can be a challenge alone.

In the preparatory discussion, we generate a differential diagnosis for the conflict situation. Generating many possible explanations keeps us curious. In Helen's case, we first identified factors in her decision-making (Box 5.3). How much could Helen understand her prognosis given her pain and delirium? Were language and cultural barriers preventing her family from hearing the low likelihood of benefit from further treatment? (This failure to hear is common and well

---

Box 5.3 **Patient and Family Factors Complicating the Discussion of Prognosis or Medical Options**

Not understanding the medical situation due to
- being emotionally overwhelmed or exhausted
- medical problems impeding understanding—hypoactive delirium, neurologic disorders
- communication barriers—medical jargon, euphemisms, or language
- insufficient time to integrate the prognosis

Avoiding discussions due to
- strong emotions—fear, anxiety, sadness, anger
- cultural or family norms

Lacking rapport with the oncologist

Confused by differing estimates of prognosis within the medical team (mixed messages)

Feeling burdened by decision-making and unable to refuse treatments

Distrusting the medical system, making it hard to accept a recommendation to stop treatment

Strongly valuing living as long as possible and trying all options

Young and wanting aggressive treatment

---

documented in the literature. In one study of patient/clinician pairs, when the clinician reported saying to the patient that the patient could die from the underlying disease, only 54% of the patients reported such a discussion.) We also thought that Helen or her family might feel obligated to accept treatment if offered, given Helen's obvious suffering.

We also identified factors in the oncologist's decision-making (Box 5.4). The oncologist and our team had a close relationship. We had shared many cases with her and trusted her judgment. What she was seeing that we were missing? Was it a medical nuance? Did family pressure or strong feelings make her backtrack when discussing the prognosis and options?

With a reasonable differential diagnosis in hand and ready to learn more, we were ready to meet.

Box 5.4 CLINICIAN FACTORS COMPLICATING THE DISCUSSION OF PROGNOSIS OR MEDICAL OPTIONS

Uncertainty about the prognosis

Uncertainty about the best treatment due to new treatments, standards of care, or clinical trials

Difficulty talking honestly with the patient about the prognosis and treatment options due to worries about taking away hope

Backtracking due to discomfort with strong patient emotions

Difficulty making recommendations due to concerns about patient autonomy

Misconception that palliative care is needed only at the very end of life

Disagreement between the oncologist and palliative care clinician about the prognosis or best treatment options

---

Talking with Colleagues

Before a difficult conversation with a colleague, we remember our pallia-tive care skills, honed over the years with patients!

Even with a colleague we know well, we start with developing rapport—whether by sitting down, asking open-ended questions, listening carefully, or spending time on nonclinical topics. Although using these skills can be difficult during a rushed clinical day or on the phone, we try anyway, even if simply by confirming that now is a good time to talk or by asking how our colleague is doing.

The goal of the conversation is to understand the oncologist's perspec-tive. This curiosity can be difficult to find when we have followed the patient for months or years and have formed opinions about the clinical situation and a connection to the patient. With curiosity in mind, we ask early in the discussion how the oncologist sees the situation. For example, in Helen's case: "I am trying to figure out how to help Helen best. Can you tell me what you are thinking about her prognosis and options for treatment?" We ask also about the patient's functional status and the likely illness trajec-tory: "Can you tell me more about what you think the next few months will be like?" Best case/worst case questions can explicate the range of the prog-nosis: "In the best case, what are you hoping for? What is the prognosis in the worst case—say, if she does not respond to treatment?"

Helen's oncologist acknowledged that immunotherapy was a long shot, but she had seen surprising responses in other patients. She knew that Helen was suffering and thought that the treatment could help. She had discussed the option with Helen and her family, who were considering it. The plan was to start the treatment in the hospital as Helen was too sick to be discharged (a warning sign that the likelihood of benefit was low).

When we still worry about the prognosis or the direction of treatment after hearing the oncologist's perspective, as in Helen's case, we honestly share our worries. As with clinical care, we can broach difficult topics honestly and respectfully using "I" statements or "I" messages. This ap-proach originates in Carl Rogers's nondirective approach to therapy and in parenting research of the 1970s. (One author was taught this method of honest communication in fifth grade.) "I" statements allow us to express feelings, beliefs, or values in a nonthreatening way by presenting the viewpoint as the opinion of one person, rather than as a fact or universal truth.

To share concerns or worries, the natural form of the "I" statement is "I worry that . . .": "I worry that Helen is dying despite our best efforts." By presenting our belief as subject to doubt, we invite a conversation. By expressing worry, we focus the conversation on our shared problem, how to care for our patient. We are saying, "I am struggling with how to help her best. I know that you are too." Our doubts can then be seen as concern for the patient, rather than as criticism of our colleague's judgment.

We can deepen alignment (now with the oncologist) by pairing our "I worry" statement with our hopes: "I too hope that the immunotherapy works. This patient has had such a rough ride with the illness. It would be so nice if she could catch a break. I also worry that, by focusing on treatment rather than comfort, we are aggravating her suffering. We haven't really controlled her pain other than by sedating her."

We structure the conversation around the clinical goals of the patient: "It's hard to know how to help her best. On the one hand, I know that she wants to get better if she can. On the other hand, I know that she does not want to suffer." (Here, we name the dilemma faced by the treatment team—that Helen has two potentially conflicting goals, to try to get better and to avoid suffering.) When we share with the oncologist the complexity of the patient's conflicting values, the whole treatment team can discuss how to incorporate these values into decision-making.

The honest discussion with Helen's oncologist helped us jointly craft a two-part plan: trying immunotherapy while maintaining her comfort. Helen would start immunotherapy in the hospital. We would manage her pain aggressively, even if doing so led to sedation or delirium, keeping her comfortable while we tried to prolong her life. But if Helen became sicker, we would stop cancer-directed treatment.

After a few weeks, Helen improved. Her pain lessened and her opioids could be reduced. Her delirium cleared, and she could even play with her grandchildren, who visited the hospital regularly. She lived for several years on immunotherapy before her cancer eventually progressed.

Our relationship with Helen's oncologist strengthened as a result of this experience. Passing in the halls, we and the oncologist still remember Helen—how sick she was, how hard it was to know what to do, and how remarkably she responded to treatment.

Helen illustrates the complexity, the frustration, and the joys of our work with oncology. With ongoing breakthroughs in cancer treatment, we see great successes. However, these treatment advances have also increased prognostic uncertainty, making medical decision-making more difficult.

MEETING THE CHALLENGE OF ACKNOWLEDGING END OF LIFE

As Helen's case shows, meeting the fifth challenge of acknowledging end of life does not require that the patient reduce or forgo treatment. Some patients will choose additional treatment, and some of these patients will experience sustained benefit and can return to the third challenge of living well with serious illness. Meeting the fifth challenge *does* require that the clinician and patient find a way to acknowledge what is happening.

The ultimate goal of helping patients take up the five challenges is to help them live and die well. Like living well, dying well is best defined by the patient. For some, it means a gentle transition to hospice. Others might prefer a cardiac arrest while sleeping. And for some, dying well means trying everything until the last minute. As one of our patients told us, "I would eat a monkey's a** if I could have more time with my son." The approach detailed in this book is not about limiting patients' choices. It is about helping patients understand and cope with illness so that they can make informed choices consistent with their values.

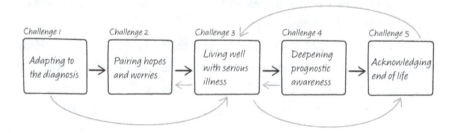

COMMUNICATION SKILLS SUMMARY

CHAPTER 1: ADAPTING TO THE DIAGNOSIS

Assess prognostic awareness: What is your understanding of your illness? Looking to the future, what are your hopes? What are your worries?

Support coping: Normalize, align, contain.

Be an interpreter: Interpret the patient for the oncologist and the oncologist for the patient.

CHAPTER 2: PAIRING HOPES AND WORRIES

For patients who focus solely on hope: Align with hope and touch upon the illness by
- empathizing
- understanding the illness's impact on others
- suggesting a worried part
- mentioning the "what ifs"
- linking to worries with "even though"

For patients who acknowledge hopes and worries: Pair the patient's hopes and worries, and normalize these mixed feelings.

CHAPTER 3: LIVING WELL WITH SERIOUS ILLNESS

Promote healthy coping by
- exploring what it means to live well with the illness
- asking how patients have coped and are coping
- introducing new skills to broaden the patient's repertoire (behavioral, cognitive, emotional, existential)

CHAPTER 4: DEEPENING PROGNOSTIC AWARENESS

For patients who can pair hopes and worries: Invite a serious illness conversation about hopes, worries, and what's important, and then complete advance directives.

For patients hesitant to talk about worries:
- Begin the conversation by aligning with or acknowledging hope and explore worries with hypothetical questions, a parts approach, or talking about talking about it.
- Continue the conversation by exploring, interpreting the patient's experience, allowing feelings to flow, and checking in.
- Close the conversation by changing topics, naming the patient's topic change, and wrapping up.

CHAPTER 5: ACKNOWLEDGING END OF LIFE

Acknowledge end of life by
- using Ask-Ask-Ask Tell Ask
- pairing hope with worry
- layering the prognostic disclosure
- naming the dilemma

Make a recommendation about treatment decisions and disposition by
- reflecting on the options
- understanding the patient's values and goals
- synthesizing a recommendation

FURTHER READING

Alfandre, D. (2016). Clinical recommendations in medical practice: A proposed framework to reduce bias and improve the quality of medical decisions. *Journal of Clinical Ethics, 27*(1), 21–27.

Back, A. L., & Arnold, R. M. (2006). Discussing prognosis: "How much do you want to know?" Talking to patients who do not want information or who are ambivalent. *Journal of Clinical Oncology, 24*(25), 4214–4217.

Back, A. L., Arnold, R. M., Baile, W. F., Tulsky, J. A., & Fryer-Edwards, K. (2005). Approaching difficult communication tasks in oncology. *CA: Cancer Journal for Clinicians, 55*(3), 164–177.

Beckman, H. B., Wendland, M., Mooney, C., Krasner, M. S., Quill, T. E., Suchman, A. L., & Epstein, R. M. (2012). The impact of a program in mindful communication on primary care physicians. *Academic Medicine, 87*(6), 815–819.

Billings, J. A. (2012). Humane terminal extubation reconsidered: The role for preemptive analgesia and sedation. *Critical Care Medicine, 40*(2), 625–630.

Billings, J. A., & Krakauer, E. L. (2011). On patient autonomy and physician responsibility in end-of-life care. *Archives of Internal Medicine, 171*(9), 849–853.

Blinderman, C. D., Krakauer, E. L., & Solomon, M. Z. (2012). Time to revise the approach to determining cardiopulmonary resuscitation status. *Journal of the American Medical Association, 307*(9), 917–918.

Campbell, T. C., Carey, E. C., Jackson, V. A., Saraiya, B., Yang, H. B., Back, A. L., & Arnold, R. M. (2010). Discussing prognosis: Balancing hope and realism. *Cancer Journal, 16*(5), 461–466.

Christakis, N. A., & Lamont, E. G. (2000). Extent and determinants of error in doctors' prognoses in terminally ill patients: Prospective cohort study." *BMJ (Clinical Research Edition), 320*(7233), 469–472.

Clayton, J. M., Butow, P. N., Arnold, R. M., & Tattersall, M. H. (2005). Fostering coping and nurturing hope when discussing the future with terminally ill cancer patients and their caregivers. *Cancer, 103*(9), 1965–1975.

Einstein, D. J., Einstein, K. L., & Mathew, P. (2015). Dying for advice: Code status discussions between resident physicians and patients with advanced cancer—a national survey. *Journal of Palliative Medicine, 18*(6), 535–541.

Einstein, D. J., Ladin, K., & Mathew, P. (2016). The ethical imperative of healthy paternalism in advance directive discussions at the end of life." *JAMA Oncology, 2*(4), 429–430.

Elwyn, G., Frosch, D., Thomson, R., Joseph-Williams, N., Lloyd, A., Kinnersley, P., Cording, E., Tomson, D., Dodd, C., Rollnick, S., Edwards, A., & Barry, M. (2012). Shared decision making: A model for clinical practice. *Journal of General Internal Medicine, 27*(10), 1361–1367.

Fried, T. R. (2016). Shared decision making: Finding the sweet spot. *New England Journal of Medicine, 374*(2), 104–106.

Fried, T. R., Bradley, E. H., & O'Leary, J. (2003). Prognosis communication in serious illness: Perceptions of older patients, caregivers, and clinicians. *Journal of the American Geriatrics Society, 51*(10), 1398–1403.

Goold, S. D., Williams, B., & Arnold, R. M. (2000). Conflicts regarding decisions to limit treatment: A differential diagnosis. *Journal of the American Medical Association, 283*(7), 909–914.

Gordon, T. (1970). *Parent effectiveness training: The proven program for raising responsible children.* Harmony Books.

Greer, J. A., Pirl, W. F., Jackson, V. A., Muzikansky, A., Lennes, I. T., Gallagher, E. R., Prigerson, H. G., & Temel, J. S. (2014). Perceptions of health status and survival in patients with metastatic lung cancer. *Journal of Pain and Symptom Management, 48*(4), 548–557.

Greer, J. A., Pirl, W. F., Jackson, V. A., Muzikansky, A., Lennes, I. T., Heist, R. S., Gallagher, E. R., & Temel, J. S. (2012). Effect of early palliative care on chemotherapy use and end-of-life care in patients with metastatic non-small-cell lung cancer. *Journal of Clinical Oncology, 30*(4), 394–400.

Halpern, S. D., Loewenstein, G., Volpp, K. G., Cooney, E., Vranas, K., Quill, C. M., McKenzie, M. S., Harhay, M. O., Gabler, N. B., Silva, T., Arnold, R., Angus, D. C., & Bryce, D. (2013). Default options in advance directives influence how patients set goals for end-of-life care. *Health Affairs, 32*(2), 408–417.

Jacobsen, J., Kvale, E., Rabow, M., Rinaldi, S., Cohen, S., Weissman, D, & Jackson, V. (2014). Helping patients with serious illness live well through the promotion of adaptive coping: A report from the Improving Outpatient Palliative Care (IPAL-OP) initiative. *Journal of Palliative Medicine, 17*(4), 463–468.

Kendall, A., & Arnold, R. M. (2008). Conflict resolution II: Principled negotiation #184. *Journal of Palliative Medicine, 11*(6), 926–927.

Kruser, J. M., Taylor, L. J., Campbell, T. C., Zelenski, A., Johnson, S. K., Nabozny, M. J., Steffens, N. M., Tucholka, J. L., Kwekkeboom, K. L., & Schwarze, M. L. (2017)."Best case/worst case": Training surgeons to use a novel communication tool for high-risk acute surgical problems. *Journal of Pain and Symptom Management, 53*(4), 711–719.

Kutner, J. S., Steiner, J. F., Corbett, K. K., Jahnigen, D. W., & Barton, P. L. (1999). Information needs in terminal illness. *Social Science and Medicine, 48*(10), 1341–1352.

Lakin, J. R., & Jacobsen, J. (2019). Softening our approach to discussing prognosis. *JAMA Internal Medicine, 179*(1), 5–6.

Nolan, M. T., Hughes, M., Narendra, D. P., Sood, J. R., Terry, P. B., Astrow, A. B., Kub, J., Thompson, R. E., & Sulmasy, D. P. (2005). When patients lack capacity: The roles that patients with terminal diagnoses would choose for their physicians and loved ones in making medical decisions. *Journal of Pain and Symptom Management, 30*(4), 342–353.

Ornstein, K. A., Aldridge, M. D., Garrido, M. M., Gorges, R., Meier, D. E., & Kelley, A. S. (2015). Association between hospice use and depressive symptoms in surviving spouses. *JAMA Internal Medicine, 175*(7), 1138–1146.

Parry, R., Land, V., & Seymour, J. (2014). How to communicate with patients about future illness progression and end of life: A systematic review. *BMJ Supportive and Palliative Care, 4*, 331–341.

Pirl, W. F., Greer, J. A., Irwin, K., Lennes, I. T., Jackson, V. A., Park, E. R., Fujisawa, D., Wright, A. A., & Temel, J. S. (2015). Processes of discontinuing chemotherapy for metastatic non-small-cell lung cancer at the end of life. *Journal of Oncology Practice, 11*(3), e405–e412.

Prochaska, M. T., & Sulmasy, D. P. (2015). Recommendations to surrogates at the end of life: A critical narrative review of the empirical literature and a normative analysis. *Journal of Pain and Symptom Management, 50*(5), 693–700.

Quill, T. E., & Brody, H. (1996). Physician recommendations and patient autonomy: Finding a balance between physician power and patient choice. *Annals of Internal Medicine, 125*(9), 763–769.

Sarela, A. I. (2013). Stop sitting on the fence: Recommendations are essential to informed decision making. *BMJ (Clinical Research Edition, 347*, f7600.

Schenker, Y., Crowley-Matoka, M., Dohan, D., Tiver, G. A., Arnold, R. M., & White, D. B. (2012). "I don't want to be the one saying 'we should just let him die' ": Intrapersonal tensions experienced by surrogate decision makers in the ICU. *Journal of General Internal Medicine, 27*(12), 1657–1665.

Schenker, Y., White, D. B., Crowley-Matoka, M., Dohan, D., Tiver, G. A., & Arnold, R. M. (2013). "It hurts to know . . . and it helps": Exploring how surrogates in the ICU cope with prognostic information. *Journal of Palliative Medicine, 16*(3), 243–249.

Sharma, R. K., Jain, N., Peswani, N., Szmuilowicz, E., Wayne, D. B., & Cameron, K. A. (2014). Unpacking resident-led code status discussions: Results from a mixed methods study. *Journal of General Internal Medicine, 29*(5), 750–757.

Stone, D., Patton, B., Heen, S., & Fisher, R. (1999). *Difficult conversations: How to discuss what matters most.* Penguin Group.

The, A. M., Hak, T., Koeter, G., & van Der Wal, G. (2000). Collusion in doctor–patient communication about imminent death: An ethnographic study. *British Medical Journal, 321*(7273), 1376–1381.

Traeger, L., Rapoport, C., Wright, E., El-Jawahri, A., Greer, J. A., Park, E. R., Jackson, V. A., & Temel, J. S. (2020). Nature of discussions about systemic therapy discontinuation or hospice among patients, families, and palliative care clinicians during care for incurable cancer: A qualitative study. *Journal of Palliative Medicine, 23*(4), 542–547.

Ubel, P. A. (2002). "What should I do, doc?": Some psychologic benefits of physician recommendations. *Archives of Internal Medicine, 162*(9), 977–980.

White, D. B., Evans, L. R., Bautista, C. A., Luce, J. M., & Lo, B. (2009). Are physicians' recommendations to limit life support beneficial or burdensome? Bringing empirical data to the debate. *American Journal of Respiratory and Critical Care Medicine, 180*(4), 320–325.

White, D. B., Malvar, G., Karr, J., Lo, B., & Curtis, J. R. (2010). Expanding the paradigm of the physician's role in surrogate decision-making: An empirically derived framework. *Critical Care Medicine, 38*(3), 743–750.

ACKNOWLEDGMENTS

This work is a collaborative project that has spanned two decades and was helped by many. Our outpatient clinic would not have come to fruition and advanced to where it is today without the visionary MGH oncology leadership past and present, Bruce Chabner, Tom Lynch, and Dave Ryan. We thank the entire palliative care outpatient clinic, especially Mihir Kamdar and Simone Rinaldi, who have built the clinic that serves as the foundation for all of our early integrated palliative care studies. Without these skilled clinicians and leaders, none of this work would have been possible. For years we have worked with these ideas and sought the guidance of our colleague David Doolittle, whose work in psychology for those with serious illness was instrumental.

We thank Michelle Seaton for her insightful development editing and encouragement. For qualitative analyses that underlie our approach we are indebted to Elyse Park. For reading versions of this manuscript we thank Daniel Shalev, Keri Brenner, Christine Ritchie, Corinne Alexander, Sharon Levine, Leah Rosenberg, and Sanjoy Mahajan. We thank Jane deLima Thomas for her tireless advocacy for structured writing and clear thinking; Sarah Rossmassler for introducing us to the idea of backcasting; Tony Back for being an inspiration, with decades of clear and thoughtful writing; and Susan Block for her mentorship and insight into psychologically informed palliative care.

Some writing was previously published in several sources. We thank the publishers for permission to adapt the following material for this book:

Jacobsen J, Thomas JD, Jackson VA. (2013). Misunderstandings about prognosis: An approach for palliative care consultants when the patient does not seem to understand what was said. *Journal of Palliative Medicine, 16*(1), 91–95. (*The Journal of Palliative Medicine* is published by Mary Ann Liebert, New Rochelle, NY.)

Jackson VA, Jacobsen J, Greer JA, Pirl WF, Temel JS, Back AL. (2013). The cultivation of prognostic awareness through the provision of early palliative care in the ambulatory setting: A communication guide. *Journal of Palliative Medicine, 16*(8), 894–900.

Jacobsen J, Kvale E, Rabow M, Rinaldi S, Cohen S, Weissman D, Jackson VJ. (2014). Helping patients with serious illness live well through the promotion of adaptive coping: A report from the Improving Outpatient Palliative Care (IPAL-OP) initiative. *Journal of Palliative Medicine, 17*(4), 463–468.

Back AL, Park ER, Greer JA, Jackson VA, Jacobsen JC, Gallagher ER, Temel JS. (2014). Clinician roles in early integrated palliative care for patients with advanced cancer: A qualitative study. *Journal of Palliative Medicine, 17*(11), 1244–1248.

Jacobsen J, Greer J, Temel J, Pirl W, Jackson VA. (2016). Stronger together: How to implement oncology and palliative care co-management. *Journal of Community and Supportive Oncology, 14*(12), 494–500.

Jacobsen J, Brenner K, Greer J, Jacobo M, Rosenberg L, Nipp R, Jackson V. (2018). When a patient is reluctant to talk about it: A dual framework to focus on living well and tolerate the possibility of dying. *Journal of Palliative Medicine, 21*(3), 322–327.

Jacobsen J, Blinderman C, Alexander-Cole C, Jackson J. (2018). "I'd recommend . . ." How to incorporate your recommendation into shared decision making for patients with serious illness. *Journal of Pain and Symptom Management, 55*(4), 1224–1230.

Traeger L, Rapoport C, Wright E, El-Jawahri A, Greer JA, Park ER, Jackson VA, Temel JS. (2020). Nature of discussions about systemic therapy discontinuation or hospice among patients, families, and palliative care clinicians during care for incurable cancer: A qualitative study. *Journal of Palliative Medicine*, *23*(4), 542–547.

Juliet Jacobsen, MD is an interventionalist for the Cancer Outcomes Research Team's palliative care studies, including the landmark *New England Journal of Medicine* study. She has worked with colleagues to define and describe the clinical work of early integrated palliative care and designed curricula for interventionalists. This has led to several peer-reviewed publications, which serve as the foundation of this book. Dr. Jacobsen has long partnered with Dr. Jackson in the intellectual work of early integrated palliative care. They have used their experiences to refine the methods by which communication around serious illness can be taught to palliative care specialists. In addition, Dr. Jacobsen has collaborated with Drs. Jackson, Greer, and Temel to develop a working model of how to study and validate the methods proposed for effective delivery of early integrated palliative care. In writing this book, Dr. Jacobsen conceptualized the five challenges faced by patients with serious illness.

Vicki Jackson, MD, MPH is a palliative care physician who, with her colleagues, has developed and refined the theoretical and clinical basis of the early integrated palliative care model by defining the intervention and establishing best practices. She has collaborated extensively with Drs. Jacobsen, Greer, and Temel to develop and validate the outcomes of integrated palliative care. As senior member of the MGH Cancer Outcomes Research team, she has been the principal palliative care investigator in numerous clinical trials of early integrated palliative care, leading the education and training of the interventionists and ensuring the fidelity of intervention delivery across study sites. She has had a deep interest in the psychological elements of palliative care and has worked closely with Dr. Jacobsen to articulate and disseminate these core clinical concepts of outpatient palliative care, which are the basis for this book.

Joseph Greer, PhD is a clinical psychologist who has worked with colleagues to evaluate the impact of the early integrated palliative care model on outcomes for patients with advanced lung cancer. This led to rigorous analyses of patient-reported data that validated the interventions designed by palliative care colleagues. He, along with Drs. Jacobsen and Jackson, developed an early integrated palliative care manual, which has been adapted for numerous clinical trials. In collaboration with Dr. Temel, Dr. Greer led the quantitative and qualitative analyses that demonstrated that one mechanism by which early integrated palliative care improves quality of life is through positive changes in patient coping skills. Dr. Greer has been a key thought partner to Drs. Jackson and Jacobsen as they have worked to further define the nuanced palliative care clinical work being done in the patient encounter. This research is highlighted throughout the book, along with a discussion of the clinical application of ways to promote adaptive coping in patients with serious illness.

When **Jennifer Temel**, MD began oncology training, palliative care was practiced exclusively in the hospital setting through inpatient palliative care consultative models or in the home with hospice care. Because palliative care interactions were often brief and intermittent and occurred late in the course of illness, many patients with serious cancers and their family members were left struggling to address their physical and psychological symptoms as well as to understand and cope with their illness. Dr. Temel worked with senior colleagues to develop, implement, and study an outpatient palliative care model that would enable patients with advanced lung cancer to receive early palliative care integrated with their oncology care. As this research platform grew, the investigative team expanded to include Drs. Jackson, Greer, and Jacobsen as well as many additional palliative care and oncology clinicians, who enabled them to further refine, understand, and study this innovative early integrated palliative and oncology care model that forms the basis for this book.

INDEX

For the benefit of digital users, indexed terms that span two pages (e.g., 52–53) may, on occasion, appear on only one of those pages.

Tables, figures, and boxes are indicated by *t*, *f*, and *b* following the page number.

Printed in the USA
CPSIA information can be obtained
at www.ICGtesting.com
LVHW021923181123
763973LV00002B/5